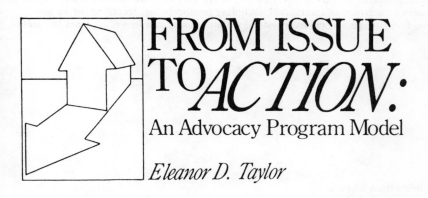

FROM ISSUE TO*ACTION:*
An Advocacy Program Model

Eleanor D. Taylor

FAMILY SERVICE
LANCASTER, PA

361.25
T213 f

Copyright © 1987 by Eleanor D. Taylor

For information address:

Family Service
630 Janet Avenue
Lancaster, PA 17601

Printed in the United States of America

FIRST PRINTING 1987

SECOND PRINTING 1991

LCCN: 91-111439

ISBN: 0-9628875-0-1

CONTENTS

LIST OF ILLUSTRATIONS

PREFACE

Although a great deal has been written on _why_ cause advocacy should be an integral part of social agencies and other human service organizations, there is less to guide the practicing advocate, and still less to guide the organization in _how_ to develop and manage an advocacy program. I became aware of this lack when we at Family and Children's Service of Lancaster County were conceptualizing our program. The need for guidelines on how to advocate became acute when we began to work on issues.

That other agencies needed these same guidelines became apparent when I taught advocacy skills to beginning advocates at the first national Family Service Association of America (FSAA) Advocacy Conference at Zion, Illinois in 1978 and at several subsequent workshops in the five-state Middle Atlantic Region of FSAA. It seemed that a manual that focused on how to develop an advocacy program and the advocacy process itself was urgently needed.

This book undertakes to meet that need by using one program as a possible model, the Family Advocacy Program at Family and Children's Service of Lancaster County, Pennsylvania. _From Issue to Action_ examines how to take the first steps in formulating an advocacy program by writing a proposal for board and staff to consider, how to deal with possible resistance through education and empowerment, how to build accountability at all levels into an advocacy program, and how people -- staff, board, community professionals and people experiencing the problem about which you are advocating -- can be empowered and involved in the advocacy effort. The book offers specifics regarding criteria for choosing issues for study and advocacy action, the various roles in the advocacy program and how to move from study of the issue to action in the advocacy effort. Finally, it shows how a guide for evaluation of the total program can be drawn up and how to build a base from which evaluation can be done effectively.

This advocacy program model is used in a largely United Way funded family service agency employing fifteen Master of Social Work caseworkers. In addition to advocacy, the agency offers programs in family counseling, family life education, adoption and teenage parenthood. In a given year over half the staff and at least half of the twenty-four board members have been actively involved in some aspect of the advocacy program. In addition, other professionals in the community and people experiencing the problem have worked shoulder to shoulder in the agency's advocacy efforts. No one had community organization experience, so that it was necessary for caseworkers to transfer their casework skills to advocacy, and for board members and others to use or develop their problem-solving skills.

Although this book shows how the Lancaster agency developed a structure that worked for them, inherent in it is the message that each organization must, as they did, think through the structure that will work best for it.

For the program model on which this book is based, I am deeply indebted to board, staff and community members of the Lancaster agency, whose combined creative thinking in countless meetings shaped the structure of the advocacy program and enriched it with guidelines as the program grew. Special mention goes to the two executives, Allen R. Smith and James Eckert, whose innovative thinking and unstinting support enabled and sustained this new program. For their assistance in reading the manuscript, providing helpful suggestions, and encouraging its completion, I am indebted to fellow advocates Wendy Puff, Trudy Brandt, Debra Meckley and James Eckert. To David Taylor and Joe Barry my appreciation for the cover design, and to Mary Moscony and Patricia Frey my gratitude for their careful typing of the manuscript. Finally, to my husband, my deep gratitude for his constant support and careful review of the manuscript.

By sharing how one model works, and the theoretical skills required to implement it, I hope that administrators of social service and other human service organizations will be encouraged and empowered to make advocacy an integral part of their service to people. In addition, I hope that caseworkers, human service professionals, board members, community leaders, and people experiencing system problems will be enabled to develop their advocacy skills and effective advocacy programs.

Eleanor D. Taylor, M.S.W.
Advocacy Coordinator

ONE

ADVOCACY: BEGINNING STEPS

You want to start an advocacy program in your organization. You are a staff member convinced about the value of cause advocacy, but not sure how it works. You are an executive who feels compelled to add advocacy because of accreditation requirements. You are a student who wants to learn about advocacy for your future work. Whatever your motivation or degree of experience in other types of programs, you need somewhere to turn to see how advocacy works, and how it might function in your particular organization. This book is an attempt to meet these needs through exploration of the development of an advocacy program and how it worked in one counseling agency, Family and Children's Service, Lancaster, Pa.

It is important to recognize at the outset that the structure and procedures developed in that agency are illustrative of one way to design and implement an advocacy program. Your organization must think through what would work best for you in your community. I hope that the fact that an agency in Lancaster, a very conservative, but caring community, was able to do effective advocacy can make you feel: "We could do it, too!"

This chapter will detail how we began.

In 1973, the Public Issues Committee of the Board of the agency undertook a study of the need for additional day care in the county. It concluded that such a need indeed existed and so reported to the Board. An issue of the Lancaster newspaper in September contained a report of the agency's monthly board meeting and that they had taken a position in support of more day care in Lancaster County. It occupied an inch of column space and appeared on the society page! There was no further outcome.

At the next meeting of the Public Issues Committee, our recently appointed executive director, Allen R. Smith, joined us. The Committee was laboring over how to use an excellent study by one of the board members of the Committee concerning the housing needs for low income families in Lancaster County. Smith saw at once that the Committee was spinning its wheels and convinced us that the way to gain traction was to turn to advocacy.

1

Smith argued that public issues committees dealt mainly with legislative issues where an agency's position could be used with legislators. This worked well. But for basic human rights or needs issues not tied to legislation, taking a position publicly was not in itself productive. Much more was needed to produce meaningful social change. Advocacy would address cause issues that go beyond legislative issues, though it could include them. Most important, the need for advocacy would spring from our case experience. Advocacy would allow us to advocate on behalf of a "class" (or group) of clients who were experiencing the same problem, he said. (Now we were beginning to understand. We were familiar with case advocacy, although not by that name. As caseworkers we had long been involved in helping an individual client or family through the bureaucracy to obtain rightful benefits or service.) Smith said he was talking about advocacy as a program that would give us the means to tackle the same cause issues faced by many clients, as well as other people not known to us. We had the basis for documentation easily available: in our counseling sessions, in our case records, and in information from the experience of other professionals in the community with their clients. It was up to us as caseworkers to become more sensitive to the systemic problems many of our clients were struggling with, he said. He began to talk about case-to-cause as a dynamic relationship between information and action. An advocacy program would make available a place to refer cause issues needing advocacy action.

Advocacy? Case to cause? Was that the direction a client and I should have taken several years earlier and so have helped many other families as well?

Mrs. B. was a 35-year old black woman with five children ranging in age from two to twelve. I made home visits to discuss her problems in parenting the eldest. She also needed to discuss her fears about her husband's imminent release from prison, since he had previously knifed her in the throat. We usually sat in her living room, but one day I happened to go with her to her kitchen and noticed a hole in the ceiling about three feet in diameter. I asked why this was. She replied in a resigned way that the shower overflowed and had caused the ceiling to disintegrate. She had asked her landlord to fix it, which he had promised to do, but never had.

I said I would call him, which I did, but after several weeks it was not fixed. I called again, but still without result. The executive director and I discussed legal advice and we explored use of an escrow account. The executive pointed out the risks for Mrs. B: the landlord might find other reasons than non-payment of rent to evict Mrs. B; with five children and on welfare, Mrs. B. would find it difficult to rent another house.   I discussed with Mrs. B the risks for her and the rewards for many other families if the landlord were forced to comply through use of the escrow account. She thought about it for a week and decided against withholding the rent.

This case is illustrative of the powerlessness of both the client and the caseworker.   The executive, too, though sympathetic to both caseworker and client, was powerless without his board behind him, and the board was never told of this client's plight.   It was just a case advocacy effort that failed.   The agency remained impotent in the face of blatant injustice!

As an agency, we had no clear way to deal effectively with case-to-cause issues. Case advocacy was often stymied or was not far-reaching enough. Position-taking might have given the agency the feeling it was facing issues, but clients' needs remained untouched!   Advocacy sounded like an answer to both case and cause.

The idea of advocacy was not new to me.   I had become interested in it five years earlier at a FSAA (Family Service Association of America (now FSA--Family Service America) Practice Institute in the Poconos. A group of us at the Institute sent a resolution to FSAA urging the development of advocacy programs in all family service agencies and asking for greater leadership from FSAA to do this. When I returned to Lancaster I talked enthusiastically about advocacy. However, nothing came of it in our agency.   Later, in 1969, FSAA sent a memorandum to all executives of FSAA member agencies. In it, Clark Blackburn, FSAA Executive Director, outlined family advocacy's potential for helping families and pledged FSAA leadership. In our agency the memo was filed away, and an advocacy program was not discussed seriously.

Thus, in 1973, when Smith asked me to write a proposal for a family advocacy program, the term advocacy was not unknown, but the content, scope and its basis in the values of the social work profession were vague.   Self-education was obviously needed. Fortunately, <u>Family Advocacy: A Manual for Action</u> (Manser, 1973) had just been published by FSAA, and numerous helpful journal articles had appeared.

THE VALUE BASE FOR ADVOCACY

Basic to consideration of development of an advocacy program in any organization is the value base on which it stands.   For social work this is embodied in the "Code of Ethics" adopted by the National Association of Social Workers in 1960, and amended in 1967. Cited are those parts of the "Code" (particularly those I have emphasized) that call for advocacy involvement.

> Social work is based on humanitarian, democratic ideals. Professional social workers are dedicated to service for the welfare of mankind, to the disciplined use of a recognized body of knowledge about human beings and their interactions, and to the marshaling of community resources to promote the well being of all without discrimination. . . .

> I regard as my primary obligation the welfare of the individual or group served, which includes action for improving social conditions.

The "Code of Ethics" is necessarily very general. Further delineation of why advocacy is integral to social work practice would be needed to convince both board and staff.

McCormick, (1970:8), in her excellent article on "Social Advocacy: A New Dimension in Social Work" expressed this well. She first quotes Gordon Hamilton: (in Kasius, 1962:34) "Social work is, perhaps the only profession in which involvement of the whole person within the whole situation is the goal and the process." McCormick goes on to say:

> The goal may be social betterment or personal development. The process calls for intervention in the literal meaning of 'interference that may affect the interests of others.' (Webster, 2nd ed.) Since advocacy is a form of interference [emphasis mine], it finds its place, quite logically, among the responsibilities of a profession committed to the kind of involvement that sets in motion the helping process and directs it toward 'the all-encompassing central goal and aspiration of social work,' namely, 'service for the welfare of mankind.'

Specifically focusing on family service agencies, Kahle (1970:370) recalled their early history of crusading for better living, working, education and welfare conditions for the poor. As "professionalism" increased, the emphasis was more on clinical (intrapsychic and interpersonal) factors than on social conditions, and casework became the "core service" of FSA agencies. Kahle says:

> Only in recent years have many of us begun to realize that we cannot concentrate only on a single social work method. . . .For our programs to be related to the needs of our clients, we must reach far beyond the present concept of casework to dealing with

some of the factors that defeat people. We must try to make society's defective systems serve the needs of the people rather than their own internal needs or the needs of special interest groups. We must use what we learn from our clients about the way the systems work or fail. . . .

The family agency really has no choice in whether it will or will not commit itself to advocacy as one of its functions. Without such a commitment, we are only partially serving our clients and the community.

In response to the imperative for social work to become involved in advocacy, Dean, (1977:370) writing more recently, argues that "social work cannot survive or maintain its credibility if it operates solely in one-to-one relationships, in small groups, or in clinical settings, and fails to deal with social forces and social policy." He suggests that social work should expend equal energy for various "practice issues and activities ranging from the helping of individuals to the changing of social systems." [emphasis mine] Dean predicts that without such intervention, the dysfunctioning becomes cumulative. He sees the social worker as uniquely equipped to assume the task of identifying social forces that cause dysfunction.

These imperatives in the social work literature served as stimulae as a proposal for a family advocacy program was drafted that would serve as a basis for discussion with board and staff.

Before discussing the content of the proposal for a family advocacy program, let me say that I am not comfortable with the term "family advocacy." It is the term used by FSA to describe "cause" advocacy programs on behalf of (and with) many families in family service agencies. I find the term "family advocacy" misleading to the non-family service community and, to some extent, to family service agencies as well. It conjures up in my mind a picture of advocating for ideal family life (mother, father and children around the fire). This is an admirable aim, but the term itself is not sufficiently inclusive of the scope of human needs that an advocacy program can address.

In this book advocacy means cause advocacy on behalf of, or with, a "class" (or group) of persons with a similar problem. Some organizations and writers use the phrase "social advocacy" (United Charities of Chicago) or "community advocacy" (Kahle, 1970:203) and Panitch, (1974:327). I prefer to use advocacy as a generic term, and use adjectives such as internal (within the organization), external (other systems) or legislative, only when necessary to clarify the particular target of the advocacy effort.

However, since our agency program is actually called Family

Advocacy in keeping with FSA guidelines, that terminology will appear at times in the text in reference to agency documents. With that terminology clarified, we can turn to the substance of our proposal for an advocacy program.

PURPOSE OF A WRITTEN PROPOSAL

A written proposal for a family advocacy program geared to existing problems, needs and goals of the agency is a useful tool to obtain beginning staff and board involvement. It provides a basis for learning and discussion of positive and negative reactions. It begins the very important process of board and staff thinking through a new program.

INITIAL PROPOSAL FOR AN ADVOCACY PROGRAM

An initial proposal needs to address the following:

Why is advocacy needed in this organization?

How would the agency advocate on an issue? (Give an example of successful advocacy in a similar agency).

What is advocacy?

How do staff and board become attuned to advocacy situations?

What is the advocacy method?

What interventions would the organization use to effect social change?

What would be the scope and limits of advocacy within the organization?

How would the organization's tax exempt status be affected?

Where would resources of time (staff and volunteer) be found for an advocacy program?

What are some alternative ways to organize an advocacy program?

What are the limitations and potentialities of an advocacy program?

A proposal for an advocacy program should be designed to inform, to exhort, and to deal with concerns.

6

Our proposal began by outlining the frustration felt by caseworkers in dealing with cause issues arising from their casework experience.

> Although as social caseworkers and board members we
> want to help our clients through social action, we have
> no agency structure through which to accomplish this.
> Taking positions as a board and staff seems to meet our
> need rather than to accomplish very much for our
> clients! Many of us have come to feel that helping
> a client adjust to a faulty system is indeed giving out
> Band-Aids when corrective surgery is what is
> indicated. Taking a stand is important, but more and
> more family service agencies are facing up to the
> challenge of becoming sufficiently knowledgeable about
> a faulty system, which demeans or denies a person's
> rights, to work to change the system.

If advocates can cause a system to change, all people served by it are helped; if modifications are made on a case-by-case basis, only one person is helped.

An example of advocacy was detailed in the proposal. This example, from Sunbeam Home and Family Service of Oklahoma City, has been used over and over by staff and board to describe what advocacy can do. (Manser, 1973:7) It made advocacy come alive and seem reasonable and achievable.

The case situation was that of a young mother (a client of the family service agency) who was forced to wait for several hours with her two toddlers in a public hospital clinic. Although the mother was on time for her 8:00 a.m. "appointment" for her four-year old orthopedically handicapped son, she and the children arrived home from the clinic tense and exhausted at 2:00 p.m.

When the mother shared her problem with the family service caseworker, the latter took the cause issue to the supervisor and the agency administration. Their Family Advocate contacted the hospital staff to ascertain how they dealt with appointments; the hospital staff confirmed the experience of the client, explained why they worked this way, and agreed to talk with representatives of Family Service and other agencies. The Family Advocate contacted other agencies and their collective experience of the effects of this clinic policy was documented. A meeting was then arranged between the agency representatives and the hospital staff members who had the power to modify the systems in question. When the hospital recognized that their policies were actually not serving the very families they were attempting to help, they carried through a thorough revision of the clinic scheduling processes. There were by-products of this advocacy effort: volunteers were used more effectively, and the ways in which the hospital waiting areas were organized and furnished improved; in addition, young physicians and others in training received a positive message about regard for the time and dignity of all patients.

This example illustrates how advocacy can work, going from case to cause. Agencies banding together with documented evidence of the problem and using appropriate confrontation can produce positive outcomes for all concerned.

Although examples are important and alive, family advocacy has to be defined conceptually. The following definition from Family Service Association of America (in Manser, 1973:3) was used to introduce the advocacy concept in the proposal, and later to educate those setting up the program.

> Family advocacy is a professional service designed to improve life conditions for people by harnessing direct and expert knowledge of family needs with the commitment to action and the application of skills to produce the necessary community change. The purpose of family advocacy services is to insure that systems and institutions with direct bearing on families work for those families, rather than against them.

> Family advocacy goals include not only improvement of existing public and voluntary services and their delivery, but also development of new or changed forms of social services. Any institutionalized service such as housing, employment, welfare, education, health care, recreation, transportation, police and courts, and social agencies, including family service agencies, may be in need of change to achieve its stated purposes in today's world. Advocacy may also aim a concerted action at the solution of common problems such as drug abuse,alcoholism, mental retardation, and abuse of civil rights, which affect many families in a community.

> Family advocacy service is needed by families at all economic levels, since it is concerned with provision of a humane social environment for all and is related to problems common to all. Priority for advocacy service should go to families, neighborhoods, and communities in the greatest jeopardy, who have suffered most acutely from the impact of racism, dehumanization, poverty, injustice, and inequality of opportunity.

The proposal went on to outline how family advocacy situations make themselves known:

Becoming attuned to family advocacy situations means a new kind of listening: listening for the dysfunctioning in the system or the social institutions and how it is affecting the family or individual rather than listening for the client's inability to adjust.

It means making a commitment as social workers to our <u>client</u> rather than to the <u>system.</u> Social workers prefer to work things out through consensus rather than to take less comfortable roles as adversaries. But, if we really believe in justice for our clients and if we really become attuned to the many dehumanizing situations in which individuals and families should not be asked to function, we gain the will and strength to work toward a healthier solution.

Many of the advocacy situations come to light where there are inadequacies, lack of programs, ineffective programs, or where programs are non-existent and clients simply "fall between the cracks." Perhaps the most important place to become attuned to advocacy is where we say: "We're sorry. We can't help you with that!"

In order to set up a family advocacy program, the proposal called for:

1. An agency structure setting up a family advocacy program

2. A board, executive and staff commitment to family advocacy as a program so that individual workers will have the agency behind them in advocacy situations

3. Time allotted for staff to develop the advocacy program

4. Board involvement in understanding the problems in a given advocacy situation; intervention of board members in some situations where their contribution would be more effective and influential than the caseworkers

5. Staff commitment to work as hard with and for families in family advocacy as they do in family casework

6. Legal consultation from an attorney prepared to handle advocacy situations

7. Board and staff orientation to advocacy and development of advocacy skills.

The proposal explained family advocacy as a <u>method</u> closely related to casework: advocacy's first task is to define the problem, get the facts through study, diagnose the problem, and decide where and how to intervene in order to bring about change (treatment). An explanation of how advocacy would work toward

9

change through assuming the good will of the system being asked to change was designed to minimize fears of board and staff that advocacy waves red flags. The focus of advocacy position-taking is rooted in the needs or rights of those who are being neglected, not in righteous criticism of an organization. Advocates need to realize that often in community advocacy they must continue to live with organizations who today might be adversaries and tomorrow allies in a different advocacy endeavor. In addition, much advocacy in family service agencies, at least, is concerned with other human service organizations that have become dysfunctional. These organizations were founded to serve people, and must be assumed to want to continue to do this when they are made aware of the practices that have become dysfunctional for their clients.

Advocacy would try to work with the offending system on the basis of a "you win:we win" approach. However, if cooperation were not forthcoming, confrontation would be used. It was stressed that in many, if not most, advocacy issues it would be necessary to join hands with others in the community who were concerned about the problem too. Coalitions could be more effective both in documenting the problem and in using their varied sources of influence.

Techniques of advocacy could include studies and surveys, expert testimony, case conferences with other agencies, inter-agency committees, educational methods, position-taking, administrative redress, demonstration projects, direct contacts with legislators and officials, coalition groups, client groups, petitions, and persistent demands short of harassment. (Sunley, 1970) It is important to use existing channels for redress, to work with a target system toward change, if that is possible, and, if not, to negotiate a solution. (See Chapter Seven for discussion of this.)

Demonstrations and protests, although in the repertoire of advocacy, could be used only as a last resort. The method of intervention employed and the level of confrontation used must relate to the plan for change. Efforts to change a state law, for example, would require a massive effort on many levels and with various methods, whereas challenging a practice of a local organization might be accomplished through meetings, pressures, client groups, and administrative redress. (Sunley, 1970)

The importance of evaluating what worked, or what did not, was stressed. Could a different strategy work better? Whether there was success or failure, the board must understand why. The importance of giving credit to all who contributed, including those in the system who changed, was emphasized.

In addition to concern about how confrontive or controversial advocacy might be, there might be concern about the agency losing its tax-exempt status. Two laws and the Office of Management and Budget (OMB) Regulations now affect a tax-exempt agency's decisions relative to influencing legislation. Eligible organizations can elect to remain under 501(c)(3) of the Internal Revenue Code, in which case their legislative activity must not be "substantial," or elect to take advantage of the Tax Reform Act of 1976 which has defined the permissible amount of legislative activities in terms of actual expenditures for two types of lobbying activities: "(1) traditional lobbying of legislatures and that of regulatory agencies and (2) grassroots lobbying--those attempts by an organization to influence the general public on matters of legislation." (Abernathy, 1976) Permissible expenditures in one tax year are defined specifically for traditional lobbying (for example, 20% of the first $500,000 and 15% of the second $500,000 of the organization's budget and so forth) and grassroots lobbying ("no more than 1/4 of the permissible expenditures of tax exempt funds".) (Abernathy, 1976) These specifics are in contrast to the 501(c)(3) caution that legislative activities must be "substantial" to bar an organization from tax-exempt status. This has never been defined. However, Manser (1976) indicates that in Seasongood v. Commissioner, 227F.2d 907 (6th Cir. 1955), it was judged that the dedication of "something less than 5 per cent of the time and effort of" an organization to legislative activity "could not be deemed 'substantial' within the meaning of the section."

In addition to these laws, OMB promulgated new rules effective May 1984 in its Circular A122, Cost Principles for Nonprofit Organizations concerning treatment of lobbying costs by nonprofit organizations receiving federal grants and contracts. The rules restrict the right of nonprofit organizations receiving any federal funds (except block grants) to use such funds to influence local, state and federal government decisionmaking. Agencies should consult the details of these rules relating to federal funds and their legal advisor. However, under these rules, even if a voluntary organization does not attempt to use federal funds to do permissible legislative activity, it must "disclose the amount of funds expended for influencing legislation, even though these funds are from private sources (charitable contributions, etc.)." (Child Welfare League of America "Legislative Link", May 14, 1984)

The above discussion is meant to highlight the current laws and regulations that are the parameters within which legislative advocates must function. It will be important for you to check with your legal consultant regarding budget limitations and specific permissible legislative activity.

You will note that although there are many restrictions on the use of federal funds for lobbying, other funds from private giving can be used within the tax laws of the Internal Revenue

11

Code and the Tax law of 1976. Moreover, the limitations on legislative advocacy in no way affects the scope of other advocacy efforts. An agency can advocate for system change, new services to fill unmet needs or rights, or for appropriate and speedy implementation of laws and regulations already in force. An agency can advocate for greater awareness of certain issues and improved methods of handling them. In fact, the vast majority of advocacy work in most agencies is not affected by these laws.

RESOURCES FOR AN ADVOCACY PROGRAM

When our proposal was written in 1973 this very important aspect was not included. The executive took the responsibility for finding staff time, and later designated my half time with the agency for coordination and work in the program. In 1973 there was some flexibility in agency budgets; today there is often none, so that it might be necessary to seek additional dollars to begin a program: through the United Way, a local or national foundation, a church or service group. Because volunteers can be used so effectively, a program can begin with small amounts of staff time, and therefore, a modest budget. You could take the stance that it is an obvious economy to help many people with the same problem, rather than one by one. A two-year pilot project could demonstrate the importance of an advocacy program and enable future funding.

Our executive also indicated from the beginning that additional people to work in advocacy would come from board and community volunteers. Some board members were skeptical; others were eager to begin. The people-power of board and community volunteers together with a staff person's ongoing guidance can mount an effective advocacy program. Advocacy skills are primarily problem solving skills that volunteers often find satisfaction in using to work on a cause. For many volunteers, advocacy can be an important outlet for their desire to help people when their current job does not provide this. For people who have experienced the particular problem about which one is advocating, it can be an excellent therapy to work through their frustration and anger by using their intimate knowledge to advocate for constructive change. Volunteers can feel deep satisfaction in achieving a new program or a more humanely run organization.

Let me return to discussion of the final portion of our proposal which set forth alternative ways to organize an advocacy program. These were taken from theoretical and actual models of various agencies as set forth by Manser. They were meant to be a guide in thinking through a possible model for the agency. These alternative models may be useful to you in thinking about the best way to organize advocacy in your organization.

12

ALTERNATIVE WAYS TO ORGANIZE
A FAMILY ADVOCACY PROGRAM

1. Form a permanent Family Advocacy Committee with responsibility to promote agency commitment and educate staff and board (Manser:21), select issues appropriate for agency action, assign priorities, and develop a plan of action by delegating implementation to individuals and other groups (a specific department or subcommittee) within the agency. (Manser:31)

2. Develop teams consisting of board members, executive, staff and community people most affected by the problem. Consultants can be added from various fields, with or without pay. (Manser:36)

3. Establish a Department of Family Advocacy, with employment of a full time social worker who would consult with staff regarding a range of cause issues that they have seen, compile illustrative case material for the Public Issues Committee, and involve staff in action. Volunteers, graduate students and indigenous workers could assist. (Sunley, 1970)

4. Create a part-time position for a family advocate. (Sunley, 1970)

5. Assign an existing staff member where budget does not permit expansion of staff. Part-time assignment could be made, as an expedient only, since conflict between the demands of a caseload and the advocacy function would be frequent and onerous for the worker. (Sunley,1970)

6. Form a Staff Committee, with the chairman bearing the responsibility for the advocacy function but delegating work to committee members. (Sunley, 1970)

7. Form an Agency or Inter-Agency Council:

   a. Agency Council: Appointment of a committee composed of board members, staff and volunteers from the community who determine areas in which the agency is to become involved in advocacy.

   b. Inter-Agency Council: Work for the creation of an Inter-Agency Council employing one full-time advocate. This would tie community agencies together as well as allow separate activity. (The example given was with four family agencies.) (Manser:70)

13

8. Appoint a five member committee of staff and administration, which would work closely with the board, other agencies and community groups. (Manser:72)

9. Form a Staff Advocacy Committee working with the Public Issues Committee:

    a. The staff advocacy specialist is selected: to take leadership and responsibility for carrying out the agency's advocacy program; to chair the Staff Advocacy Committee and to be the liaison between staff, board and community organizations.

    b. The Staff Advocacy Committee, with a minimum of three staff members, would serve as staff representatives on the Public Issues Committee and gather and screen information from the staff for appropriate issues to recommend to the latter committee.

    c. The Public Issues Committee is composed of board, Staff Advocacy Committee members and staff advocacy specialist. This committee reviews issues and selects those for action, develops a plan of action and assigns responsibilities; the chairman of the Public Issues Committee takes its recommendations to the Board for discussion and approval. (Manser, 1973: 78)

Which of these might work for your agency?

1. Family Advocacy Committee?

2. Advocacy teams: executive, board, staff and community people?

3. Department of Family Advocacy with a full-time staff person?

4. Part-time family advocate?

5. Existing staff member assigned to advocacy?

6. Staff committee on advocacy?

7. Agency Council or Inter-Agency Council?

8. Five member committee of staff and administration?

9. Staff Advocacy Committee working with Public Issues Committee?

The potentialities and limitations of an advocacy program are dealt with in detail in the next chapter.

In summary, the writing of a proposal has several positive aspects, which can be applied in other advocacy endeavors. (In this case it was, of course, to advocate for a family advocacy program.) First, when a request is written down, it shows that it is serious; second, it gives the writer(s) an opportunity to think through the request as clearly as possible, to research the literature, to marshal telling arguments and to establish legitimacy; third, if given to the readers in plenty of time, it gives them an opportunity to think through the various aspects and the legitimacy of the proposal; fourth, all persons considering the proposal begin from the same basic document. (See Bibliography for references that can be used as a tool in learning about advocacy, its roots in the social work professions, and how advocacy interacts and enriches other programs in an agency.)

Let me share now how staff and board reacted to the proposal.

STAFF AND BOARD REACTION

Staff reacted to discussion of the proposal without great enthusiasm, but with a modest: "Go ahead; let's see what you come up with." Staff members were already trying to adjust to the many changes made by the new executive in his first four months. They were unsure whether they wanted this new program, and perhaps, unsure how it would affect them.

In contrast, members of the Board reacted with enthusiasm, though not without many questions. They, no doubt, saw that advocacy was going to involve them in actual work on issues as well as in key policy decisions; this might have made them anticipate that they would become more involved in the work of the agency, as in fact they did. In any event, at its January meeting in 1974, the Board showed interest in the proposal and set up an ad hoc committee to study the feasibility of adopting an advocacy program. (We will look at how an advocacy program was designed by this committee in Chapter Three.)

Before moving on to Chapter Two take a moment to think about your own agency resources and the feasibility of an advocacy program in your organization.

STOP AND **THINK**

KEY ASPECTS FOR CONSIDERATION IN BEGINNING AN ADVOCACY PROGRAM

1. Who in your organization is convinced about the value of advocacy? Meet to discuss and empower one another.

2. Identify advocacy program resources (people and dollars).

3. Inform yourself and others who are interested about advocacy.

4. Write a proposal defining advocacy and setting forth the "why" and "how", giving an example of successful advocacy such as the Oklahoma example in this chapter or the shelter for abused women described in Chapter Three.

5. Set up a task group of board, staff and community people to design your advocacy program. What skills, experience and representativeness will you need to look for among staff and community? Jot down the names and what they could offer.

Name   Reason for Choice
                        (Commitment, influence,
                        expertise, experience,
                        etc.)

One

NOTE

1. Family service agencies were expected to have a board committee that focused on "community concerns or public affairs" under the requirements for membership in FSAA in 1972. Advocacy activities in agencies were encouraged, but not expected in order to meet accreditation standards, as is true at present. (See "FSAA Requirements for Membership, 1980.")

REFERENCES

ABERNATHY, J. (1976) "'76 Tax Reform Act Defines Guidelines for Lobbying by Tax-Exempt Organizations." Monitor: 2.

Child Welfare League of America (1984) Legislative Link (May).

DEAN, W. (1977) "Back to Activism." Social Work 22:370.

HAMILTON, G. (1962) "The Role of Social Casework in Social Policy," p. 34 in C. Kasius (ed.) Social Casework in the Fifties. New York: FSAA.

KAHLE, J. (1970) "Relevant Agency Programs for the Large Urban Community." Social Casework 51:202.

MANSER, E. (ed.) (1973) Family Advocacy: A Manual for Action. New York: FSAA.

McCORMICK, M. (1970) "Social Advocacy: A New Dimension in Social Work." Social Casework 51:8.

PANITCH, A. (1974) "Advocacy in Practice: From Case to Cause." Social Casework (June).

SUNLEY, R. (1970) "Family Advocacy: From Case to Cause." Social Casework (June).

BUILDING COMMITMENT

As you begin talking about an advocacy program in your agency or writing a proposal, you are, in fact, advocating for advocacy! If you are the decision-maker, you may be fully, or only partially, convinced. If you are a staff member concerned about starting an advocacy program, you will need to be sensitive to the climate in your agency and your executive's feelings. If you are a board member eager to start an advocacy program, it might be important to ally yourself with other board members to convince whoever needs convincing. However, if you are not sure about the prospect of an advocacy program, you could talk with the executive, read articles and talk with some experts in the field.

In most agencies where advocacy is discussed there will be a combination of "Yes, we can" and "No, we can't". Some people will feel empowered to do what is being asked; others will react negatively or with some resistance. In your own organization you will find some of the same resistances to change that will be evident when you begin to advocate outside your organization on some community issue. Resistance is partly fear, partly lack of knowledge and partly the fact that they have never tried it. The other side of resistance is empowerment. Obviously, empowerment is feeling free to tackle something new, untried and difficult. Since these are such basic issues in advocating for a cause or advocating for advocacy itself, let us look at how to deal with them.

RESISTANCE

At its root, resistance comes from fear: fear of the new and untried ("Advocacy makes me feel uneasy."); fear of asserting one's rights or the agency's rights ("Do we have the right to question the way that a system offers service?"); fear of questioning those in power or the status quo ("You can't fight City Hall!"); fear of retribution ("We might lose our funding or create bad feelings.").

COMMON RESERVATIONS AND FEARS OF DECISION-MAKERS ABOUT ADVOCACY

The following are some typical anxieties that decision-makers might have about embarking on an advocacy program, followed by answers that the advocate might give.

18

"To get involved in advocacy is to be too controversial."

Advocacy might be controversial, but it does not have to be. An organization can make the choice about what it works on, beginning, possibly, with the less controversial issues until it feels secure in its advocacy role.

"I do not want to march on City Hall!"

"Marching on City Hall" is the type of confrontation that would be decided on only as a last resort. Advocacy's chief intervention is dialogue and negotiation. The aim is to work with the system, if possible.

"I am afraid we would lose our funding source. The United Way would be afraid of the repercussion on givers."

A great deal of advocacy that is not controversial can be achieved. This will enhance the reputation and visibility of an agency, and therefore possibly increase giving to the United Way because the community appreciates an agency that comes to grips with community problems.

"Advocacy raises red flags!"

Advocacy need not be inflammatory. It is important for an agency to recognize that it must "live" in a community. Therefore, a better approach might be to work with the offending system, offering to work together on solutions. Then, if the target system does not change, let community pressure (actual or potential) induce change.

"Someone else can do it better. Our job is counseling."

Maybe, but family service agencies have a unique knowledge base of what families struggle with at a system level. The motto of family service agencies is: "Strength to families." Surely, this includes advocacy.

"I would hate to start something whose final result I could not foresee."

This is scary. It is also challenging. The study-action method of responsible problem solving provides a framework within which to work, plus the ideas and commitment of many people. (See Chapters Six and Seven.) Together the advocate group decides on its goals. These may have to be modified during actual negotiation, but the group will have decided together on a "fall back" position. It is better to accomplish something than not to try at all.

On the other hand, it is always possible to stop working on an issue for valid reasons. Again, this would be the joint decision of the advocate group. (See Chapter Seven.)

"Sometimes advocacy has a negative feeling to me. I don't want to appear to be an agitator or a policeman looking for trouble in another system."

No. Such a negative role is often unproductive. Advocacy seeks to bring problems into awareness: first, to assess for ourselves as advocates the extent of the problem; second, to learn from others who are concerned and knowledgeable about the issue; and third, to discuss with the offending system, our concerns and potential solutions.

The means of change can be: the system's own decision (not realizing the problem it created for those it was trying to serve), acceptance of an offer from the advocates to work with them toward system change, and if necessary, finally, confrontation or exposure in the community of a situation needing change. (See Chapter Seven.)

"As only one agency, I am sure that we would be powerless to effect any meaningful change."

Sometimes one agency can do a great deal with documentation of the problem from its caseworkers and with the backing and participation of its board and other community volunteers.

Greater power does come from agencies joining together to document problems and to demand and work for change. However, it takes one agency with advocacy skill and determination to convene a meeting of community agencies and organizations and to empower them to work for change.

"I don't like change." (Executive, supervisor, staff member.)

Change is difficult, even risky, but, if the agency's response to "families under stress" is better, you will get the credit.

20

"Won't we lose our tax-exempt status?"

No.   (See Chapter One.)

"Our Board would not 'buy' advocacy."

Try involving the Board with the staff in setting up an advocacy program. Let the Board know that it will have ultimate control. In many agencies where board members are involved in doing advocacy as well as sanctioning it, they report a feeling of greater involvement and understanding of the agency's work in all program areas.

"Staff are not interest in advocating."

Maybe some are not, but, given orientation and training, some are. Those who do involve themselves in advocacy need to be given credit for their time so spent. This might involve new statistical categories to identify time spent in advocacy as compared to counseling and other programs. If advocacy is expected as a part of a caseworker's job description, evaluation guidelines can reflect and encourage this. If no one currently on staff has the commitment or skills to do the advocacy that is needed, this would be something to look for when a new staff member is hired.

"Staff is too busy. There is already a waiting list for counseling. Staff feels that advocacy will take time from counseling."

Desch (1980) a former board president, says:

As a board we had to struggle with the reality that in order to begin an advocacy program--that is, commit staff time, which means commit agency dollars--we may have to give up something else. What would happen if clients who needed our counseling services would have to go on a waiting list in order to free staff time for an advocacy program? You'll need to address that question because, unless you plan to add staff, that's reality. We came to the conclusion that those people reached through an advocacy program needed to be served just as much as those clients who are seen in a counseling program; there is a real sense in which those persons whose needs are not met [by advocacy] are already on a waiting list.

"We have no staff with time to take on the advocacy role. We would have to hire someone, and where can I find the money?"

Begin with part time. Try to get money from a local foundation interested in beginning new programs. Since so much advocacy can be done with the help of volunteers, it can be "sold" to a funding source as relatively inexpensive, considering the number of people helped. It is also more efficient to help <u>many</u> people through a cause approach than one-by-one with case advocacy.

Discuss the situation with United Way. If advocacy solves problems, that means a better community; this is furthering United Way's goal, and makes its allocation of funds look good.

"We don't know anything about advocacy."

Get training. Send relevant staff to conferences; use the literature (see Bibliography) and obtain consultants.

"Advocacy is not 'new.' We have been doing case advocacy for years!"

Case advocacy is not new, but <u>cause</u> advocacy <u>is.</u>

1. Cause advocacy arises from the case situation (or community knowledge), and goes on to document the problem in many other situations.

2. Cause advocacy serves many people with the same problem by taking a stand for what is theirs by right from a system.

3. Cause advocacy will go beyond consensus planning to confrontation for change, if necessary.

4. Cause advocacy works with and empowers the people who are hurting from the system problem. It either empowers inadequately served people to work on their problem as a united group to obtain what they need from the system, or it joins people who are hurting with influential citizens and professionals to work toward the same goal.

"Advocacy is really just 'manipulating the environment' that caseworkers have done for years."

The . . . concept of 'manipulating the environment' leads a worker to call a worker in another institution and arrange for a personal favor. The result is often paternalistic treatment for a client, because the other worker respects 'us' -- the social worker, not the client. In Advocacy, the request is made or demanded because the person(s) or family(ies) have a right to the service. The request, demand, or whatever is necessary is made and carried through on a policy-making level. As a result, other people, known and unknown to our agencies, present and future, can and will benefit by the change. (Riley, 1971)

"Members of our casework staff say that they are upset about how some clients suffer because of their poverty and housing; they feel that these clients are dehumanized, but they don't feel they can do anything about it."

It is not only the clients who are dehumanized; case-workers who accept what they feel powerless to change are dehumanized too! An agency advocacy program could change that by being a resource for both clients and caseworkers.

As is evident from the foregoing, it is essential when advocating for advocacy to be sensitive to the very real anxieties that decision-makers might have in thinking about undertaking an advocacy program. The staff member who is interested in promoting advocacy in his/her agency might find Patti's (1974) paper on "Organizational Resistance and Change: The View from Below" helpful in understanding the dynamics within an agency (or other organization) that promote or militate against change.

Resistance might be expressed as open fear or hostility to this new idea of advocacy, or it might be expressed in apathy and indifference. However it shows itself, it will be important to recognize that some resistance to change is normal. Change in any organization, as in an individual, is unsettling and even threatening.

Since advocacy will require assertiveness from the agency as an organization and from individuals (board and staff) working in the program, some might feel less comfortable than others with this. All can be expected to feel some anxiety and to require assurance that advocacy is needed and that they have a right to do it. I will discuss the latter shortly.

Richan and Rosenberg (1971) suggest that one of the major enemies of the social worker advocate is the assumption that he will get a negative response from the target system. They suggest advocates need to "prepare for the worst by expecting the best." Not only does the advocate need to be prepared to help the target system "save face", he/she must also be ready to help the system supply a rationale for a positive response. Although systems and administrators often appear difficult to move, they are actually very sensitive to criticism and will go to great lengths to avoid trouble. Thus, they are often much more ready to say "yes" than might be expected. Assuming the best, but preparing for negative reactions is equally important in your own organization.

If you expect that resistance (fear) is normal and needs to be alleviated, you can use your power of diagnosis and human relations skills to assess the reasons for concern and deal with it, whether in your own or another system. (See Chapter Seven for discussion of dealing with resistance in other systems.) A common social work maxim that "all growth is painful" certainly applies here. As in therapy, understanding why a change is needed, why people feel as they do, and then taking time to work this through in a full discussion of positive and negative feelings should alleviate this problem to some degree. (Empowerment, which we discuss shortly, is an obvious need as well.) Clearly, it is important to recognize that many professionals prefer to stay with what they know best, or the power position they are in currently, rather than risk something new. As an advocacy program begins it appears to be typical to find a few staff who are enthusiasts, most relatively indifferent or ready to be persuaded, and a very few who are skeptical or hostile. It is important to remember, too, that a few people will never be able to advocate, either because of their value system or their passive personalities. To some extent advocates are "born", not "made."

We have looked at why fear plays such an important part in deterring the potential advocate. Now let us look at how to deal with that through a better understanding of the basis for advocacy and why advocacy is important as one aspect of an agency's work.

UNDERSTANDING THE BASIS FOR ADVOCACY

The basis for advocacy is found in our national heritage of the dignity and worth of every human being and the legal and moral rights to which each is entitled. This heritage is translated into concern for specific needs depending on the political climate at a given point in history. In the sixties and seventies the climate of the country encouraged vindication of the rights of the powerless. This was exemplified in consumer advocacy, the Civil Rights movement, the Women's Liberation movement and among the poor and hitherto invisible, in, for example, the Welfare Rights Organization and the National Association for Retarded Children. This climate for change continues; more people, such as the handicapped and the aged, who were once powerless, are banding together to gain power from their numbers and the inherent justice of their cause.

In order to feel convinced about the need for an advocacy program, each organization or profession must look to its own value base and traditions. Social work has done this as it responded to the climate of the sixties and rediscovered its roots professionally. Let us look at the social work literature to see how advocacy has come to be seen as integral to serving people.

ADVOCACY AS AN INTEGRAL PART OF SERVICES TO PEOPLE

Cooper (1977:361) sees the social work profession as "the conscience of the community" standing as it does "at the boundary of how things are and how they can become. We are, by the diverse nature of our work, history, sanctioned relationship to society, and values, uniquely capable of moving from case to cause."

Agencies need to become multidimensional rather than one-dimensional; they must not only provide service, but also take seriously their responsibility to deal with public policy, dysfunctioning systems and unmet needs. Most writers urge a balanced or holistic approach to the services that should flow from our basic social work values. One should not be given up for the other, but rather "the mission of social work [should not be] bound to the specifics of method [casework, group work or community organization], but to changing individuals, institutions and policies." (Dean, 1977:373) Family Service America expects that in addition to family counseling, hitherto considered the main function of a family service agency, its member agencies develop family life education and family advocacy. This emphasis represents the continuum from crisis through prevention to identification and work on cause issues.

Some family service agencies have found that an agency planning process forced them to recognize their purpose was to develop programs that would strengthen family life, not solely to provide a casework program for crisis situations because that was what they were trained to do. To set up new programs such as advocacy and family life education meant training, development of new skills, much risking and many growing pains. However, such agencies say that they feel that they are much more relevant to families and to their community.

Sherry (1970), speaking of the role of voluntary agencies in general, says that "their role is not primarily to serve as alternate to government, but instead, to help keep government honest and responsible. The primary role of voluntary associations in American life is to continually shape and reshape the vision of a more just social order, to propose programs which might lead to the manifestation of that vision, to argue for them with other contenders in the public arena, and to press for adoption and implementation. For voluntary associations to do less than that is to abdicate their civic responsibility."

It is equally essential when thinking about an advocacy program to be clear about advocacy's potentialities and limitations in implementing the values for which a profession stands.

IMPLEMENTATION OF PROFESSIONAL VALUES THROUGH ADVOCACY

Potentialities

Used as a method of helping people to change institutions, develop new services and assert long-withheld rights, advocacy has tremendous potential.

1. Advocacy can get at root causes, rather than, as in casework, ameliorating problems. Blackburn (in Manser, 1973:61) expressed this well.

Advocacy is systematizing for every family in your community the availability of prevention or cure of the problem you saw in that one family. Advocacy is, after finding the way to help one family, establishing a system that will get that same kind of help to every family who needs it whether they get to your office or not. Even when the systems are working we still find families or individuals who because of internal problems cannot use them effectively. So we move from case to cause and back to case. Advocacy enables and extends casework; it extends the boundaries within which caseworkers see and treat pathology.

2. Advocacy is a resource for caseworkers. If there is an advocacy program, they can log the issue with which they see clients struggling, and with which they cannot deal in the casework situation. Counselors can work on the cause issue with the advocate group and they can suggest clients who would be able to bring their experience to the advocacy effort.

3. Advocacy can involve people in their own cause issues, which in itself can be ego-building and empowering. It provides an appropriate channel for constructive use of anger about an injustice and thus becomes not just a benevolent effort on behalf of people (although that might sometimes be the only way it can operate), but better, a way to work in alliance with those who are suffering. Best of all, is the situation in which advocacy empowers people to advocate for themselves.

26

4. Advocacy can work for all segments of a community and for society as a whole. It is needed by families at all socioeconomic levels, since it relates to problems that any or all families might have. Many issues, such as abused children, abused women, the lonely aged, the divorced, know no distinctions of class, race, religion or income group. However, advocacy work should give priority to those issues that seem most pressing in any given community or at a given time in society, and should focus on those who are suffering most from dehumanization, racism, poverty, injustice and inequality of opportunity.

5. An agency's advocacy stance can provide hope to families: it can be a place for them to turn with questions regarding protection of their rights and how to deal with systems on a case or cause level.

6. Perhaps the greatest potential for advocacy is the recognition by the community (people and organizations) that here is an agency that is willing to face the issues that others see too, but feel powerless to confront. This can also encourage and empower other community organizations to be less complacent and to advocate for their constituents, to suggest coalitions, or to ask for training in advocacy skills.

7. Cause advocacy, which serves many clients, is both more efficient and more effective than case advocacy, which serves one client at a time.

Limitations

Although there is the climate for advocacy and the social work profession sees advocating as essential, it will take time for advocacy to be legitimatized in agencies generally and in schools of social work. It will take agencies doing it, people writing about it, and schools teaching what practice has found to be true, desirable and workable. Agencies who are in the forefront of such work will find it exciting and challenging, but sometimes painful and sometimes lonely.

The most significant limitation of advocacy is obvious: no agency or community or even a whole society can do everything! Advocacy leads to other advocacy: as one rock is turned over, not one problem, but many, are evident. The tasks of evolutionary change are multiple and seemingly never ending. It is, therefore, extremely important not to set out to change society, but rather to be what Miller (in Dudley, 1978:38) calls "incrementalists" who seek small cumulative gains. "The incrementalist begins with the present situation and projects short-range goals that are based on a realistic course of action rooted in real-life or existing situations." What comes back to me here is the plea of someone in our first orientation workshop for advocacy with board and staff, when small groups were asked to give their four best hopes for advocacy, and their four worst fears. One person's hope was that we "do one small thing!"

If goals are limited and reasonable, and the number of issues taken on within the capacity and time of agency staff and board to handle, chances of success on some are good. We need to remember that as caseworkers we see a lot of families about various problems: we do not expect to help all marriages or families that we see to function happily, but we try to help people make changes that will enable more satisfactory relationships. We do not always succeed, but that does not mean that we do not try with the next family who comes to us, or that we do not have conviction that our skills are good and our counseling service necessary. Similarly in advocacy, we will win some and we will lose some. The test is whether the overall advocacy effort has produced system changes and helped people!

EMPOWERMENT

To feel empowered to advocate, we must feel both ethically comfortable with the right to advocate and convinced that we can develop a power base sufficient to the task.

WHAT GIVES US THE RIGHT TO ADVOCATE?

1. The legitimacy of the cause. Legitimacy is established through documentation of the problem or through people who have experienced the problem asserting this.

2. The legal, moral or constitutional rights of the client(s) and other persons experiencing the problem.

3. The ethical code of the profession. In the case of social work this is the Code of Ethics (see Chapter One).

WHERE DO WE GET THE POWER?

The power of advocacy springs from a deeply held conviction of the dignity and worth of every human being and his or her right to the best possible life; advocacy power becomes harnessed and usable when advocacy skills come together in a vigorous alliance to work on an issue.

Nearly everyone has more power than he utilizes or perhaps realizes. Power, like muscles, requires exercising in a planned, controlled way to realize its potential, and, like muscles, can also be overstrained and used up. There is power in social work and social agencies. It must be used, used judiciously, and not thrown around; to let it

28

lie fallow in the face of the needs of those with less power would be a betrayal of our basic purposes. (Riley, 1971)

Douglas Biklen (1974:86), in his excellent book, Let Our Children Go, asserts, too, that everyone has power. He likens power to a pyramid where the person at the top is seen as powerful and people at the bottom feel that they have little power. What they do not realize is that it takes a lot of "little" people to hold up the person(s) in power at the top. Biklen reminds us that "each of us acts as a source of power for those who are higher on the pyramid than ourselves." (Emphasis added.) What we forget is that power that can be given can also be taken away. Furthermore, "institutions are the means for exercising power and not its source." (Biklin, 1973:6) (Emphasis added). Biklen suggests flattening the power pyramid by letting those in power know that you are withdrawing support or compliance and why you are doing so. By intervening in the target system through questioning decisions, making demands, or asking for a dialogue between system heads and your advocacy group, you are using one of many interventions that may threaten the target system's power and open the way for change.

How does the advocate group itself gain power? Power comes from:

1. The right to advocate (described earlier).

2. The avowed purpose and prestige of the agency to serve people through advocacy, as well as the sanction of the board for a particular cause.

3. The development of a power base by joining with others who have experienced the problem or those who feel strongly about the problem and who operate from the same moral base. (See 1. The right to advocate, above) Power comes from groups in alliance with one another. As indicated earlier, power can be gained "through a process of entering (and withdrawing from) power relationships more consciously." (Biklen, 1973:25) Numbers show the strength behind your cause and give advocates themselves a feeling of greater power and support.

4. A thorough study and planning process that

    a) studies the problem and the system in which it occurs and seeks innovative solutions to the problem.

    b) plans effective strategy interventions and makes the case for change. This will involve an awareness of change processes and how to facilitate change. (Note the similarity in casework where the caseworker must have a capacity to listen, diagnose strengths, limitations, and the capacity for change, and to deal with resistance to change.) Skill in making the case will also involve disciplined use of feelings, for example, the advocate's own anger, as well as knowing how to recognize and deal constructively with the anger of people in the target system.

5.   A reputation for successful advocacy.

6.   The target system's fear of a worse situation (for example, racial riots, disturbed children acting out in school, parents demonstrating at a school board meeting.)

ADVOCATING FROM STRENGTH

If the advocacy group moves into a discussion or confrontation with a feeling of power for all the reasons previously cited, it will be able to move from strength. It will not have to put the target system on the defensive, but rather seek its help in solving the problem. As much as possible, the advocate group needs to move in with a win:win stance: that is, we-win--and-they-win, not a we-win-and-they-lose, although sometimes that might happen, and definitely not we-lose-and-they-win, or we-lose-and-they-lose!

Advocacy, as discussed here, is _activist_ but not radical. If you are advocating from a community agency your advocacy program must remain viable in a community that supports other services of the agency, such as counseling, adoption, family life education. Advocacy does not wave red flags, but rather enters into dialogue or confronts with the aim of working together on a problem either initially or ultimately. The aim is to make the legitimacy of the cause so clear that the community will force change if the system remains adamant. If dialogue is ineffective, confrontation _might_ be necessary. See an expanded discussion of this in Chapter Seven.

However, there are times when apathy of a community, for example, defeats by passive resistance, or the resources of the advocate group are insufficient to warrant pursuit of some goals. Advocate groups do have to recognize that they cannot do everything but that they can do some things! Also, advocates must gain perspective: if not this year, maybe next year. Advocacy is a dynamic process: opportunities open up, skills increase and change might take place later rather than sooner! John W. Gardner, (1969:30) formerly of "Common Cause,", a veteran advocate, says:

30

Life never was a series of easy victories (not even a series of hard victories). We can't win every round or arrive at a neat solution to every problem. But driving, creative effort to solve problems is the breath of life, for a civilization or an individual.

Before we move to the next chapter to look at how our advocacy program was designed, think about how what we have discussed regarding resistance and empowerment would relate to your agency.

STOP AND THINK

Who will be your allies in considering an advocacy program?

What are the reasons advocacy could work in your community? In your agency?

What obstacles will you encounter in your staff? Board? Community professionals and citizens?

Consider three ways that you could build commitment to advocacy in your agency.

1.

2.

3.

REFERENCES

BIKLEN, D. (1973) "Power to Change." Syracuse University.
Center on Human Policy. Unpublished paper: 6.

BIKLEN, D. (1974) Let Our Children Go. Syracuse: Human Policy
Press.

COOPER, S. (1977) "Social Work: A Dissenting Profession."
Social Work 22:361.

DEAN, W. (1977) "Back to Activism." Social Work 22:373.

DESCH, S. and E.D. Taylor (1980) "Getting an Advocacy Program
Started." Unpublished paper. Presented at Family Service
Association of America Middle Atlantic Regional Council
Meeting.

DUDLEY, J.R. (1978) "Is Social Planning Social Work?" Social
Work 23:38.

GARDNER, J.W. (1969) No Easy Victories. New York: Harper &
Row.

MANSER, E. (ed.) (1973) Family Advocacy: A Manual for Action.
New York: Family Service Association of America.

PATTI, R.J. (1974) Organizational Resistance and Change: The
View from Below. Social Service Review 48: 367-383.

RICHAN, W.C. and M. ROSENBERG. (1971) The Advo-kit. A Self-
administered Training Program for the Social Worker Advocate.
Unpublished. Temple University, Philadelphia.

RILEY, P.V. (1971) "Family Advocacy: Case to Cause and Back to
Case." Child Welfare (July).

SHERRY, P.H. (1970) "America's Third Force." Journal of Current
Social Issues (July).

THREE

DESIGNING AN ADVOCACY PROGRAM

Let us assume that you have written a proposal for an advocacy program and that your board has agreed to set up a committee to look into the feasibility of an advocacy program in your agency.

Let us assume further that you have chosen an able committee, representative of your board and staff and knowledgeable community advocates, to design your program. What would you and your committee need to consider to complete this task?

Here are some common questions:

1. Since beginning advocates will almost certainly have differing views of what advocacy is, how can the committee come to a common view?

2. Since your advocacy program should "fit" with your agency and your community, what special considerations should be kept in mind in setting up an advocacy program? Constraints? Supports?

3. Which of the alternative ways of setting up a program outlined in Chapter One, or the model to be discussed shortly, would work best in your agency? Perhaps it will be your own "mix" of a number of these models that will work best.

4. Can you get the support of your major funding source or some alternate funding to finance the program?

5. How will you recruit, select and train advocates?

Let me address these areas by illustrating from the experience of the ad hoc Committee on the Feasibility of an Advocacy Program.

The Committee to Study the Feasibility of an Advocacy Program was made up of seven board members (Public Issues Committee (2), Casework Policy Committee (2), at-large (2) and the President), two staff members (a supervisor and me, a family caseworker), one community volunteer knowledgeable about consumer advocacy, and the executive director. The Public Issues Committee Chairman (a board member) chaired the ad hoc committee. The Committee began its work in January 1974 and worked diligently for four months. Finally, in May, it received

33

the enthusiastic support of the Board for the program definition and the structure it devised. I mention this only to point out that it takes time to design a program with which everyone feels comfortable and a program that will work in your community.

Since the term "advocacy" was poorly understood by many of the Committee, the first task was to define advocacy for the agency. The second was to design a structure through which the program could operate within the agency, and that would be considered responsible advocacy by the community. (By "community" I mean the clients and "friends of Family and Children's Service", the United Way, the agency's major funding source, other professionals, and all those who are aware - or would be - of what the agency does).

DEFINING ADVOCACY

Arriving at a definition for advocacy proved to be a difficult task that took three committee meetings. Although this seemed very time consuming, it was, in fact, time well spent, since staff and board were coming to terms with their different views of cause advocacy, particularly its differentiation from public issues, social action and case advocacy.

To assist in arriving at a definition, a subcommittee prepared the folowing definitions from which to work:

1. Webster's Dictionary (1971) defines advocacy as: "the action of advocating, pleading for, or supporting."

2. FSAA's definition (Manser, 1971:3): Family Advocacy is professional service designed to improve life conditions for people by harnessing direct and expert knowledge of family needs with the commitment to action and the application of skills to produce the necessary community change. The purpose of family advocacy services is to insure that the systems and institutions with direct bearing on families work for those families, rather than against them." (See complete FSAA definition in Chapter One.)

3. From a committee member: "Advocacy is a process or technique of bringing together internal and external forces to alter those systems and/or institutions that interfere with families and/or individuals achieving their maximum potential."

4. From Clark Blackburn, General Director of FSAA in his December 30, 1969 memorandum to executives (Manser, 1973:61):

34

Advocacy . . . is closely related to many of our present activities. Our knowledge base comes from our work with thousands of individual families, our skill is in helping them mobilize their own strengths. Advocacy is doing something about . . . causes. Advocacy is systematizing for every family in your community the availability of prevention or cure of the problem you saw in that one family. Advocacy is, after finding the way to help one family, establishing a system that will get that same kind of help to every family who needs it, whether they get to your office or not.

The Committee definition finally became:

Advocacy is a service of this agency whose goal is to fulfill human potential by improving life conditions of people. Arising primarily from case experience of unmet needs, advocacy moves from case to cause, to change dysfunctional community institutions and systems to insure that they work for people rather than against them.

(Note that "system" is broadly defined here to encompass an organization, a community, a legislature, a profession or any body of people who operate as a system.) In many instances, in addition to systemic problems, caseworkers and board members have pointed out needs or rights that were being ignored. (The agency's 1980 definition of advocacy and the Advocacy Program goals and objectives are set forth in Chapter Four).

(It might be helpful to refer to a longer definition adopted in 1978 by the Family Advocacy Network, a group of staff advocates from family agencies in the U.S. and Canada, whose goal is to encourage family advocacy programs in all family service agencies. See Appendix 1).

What was important in the Committee's work of defining advocacy in 1974 was the process through which they (and later other agency board, staff and community volunteers) educated themselves to what advocacy is. Defining is a means of learning; it is also a means of coming to a baseline of understanding.

ADVOCACY IN THE AGENCY AND COMMUNITY CONTEXT

When one has decided what advocacy is, it is extremely important to consider the community context within which the agency will attempt to carry out this program. It is equally important to be aware of the context within the agency. Let me introduce you to Lancaster and the Family and Children's Service agency to illustrate how particular factors in a community and in an agency impinge on how advocacy needs to be designed. I will

35

also note the support (or the reverse) that those factors can be.

Lancaster is a city of 54,700 people set in the rolling countryside of Lancaster County, Pennsylvania. It is called "The Garden Spot", not undeservedly, since farming is still the way of life for many; however, after taking into account Armstrong, who has its headquarters and plant here, light manufacturing is probably the chief industry. The County has a population of some 362,346 people and is now mainly suburban. Its values are deeply rooted in the family, the church, and conservative politics. Mennonite, Amish, Scots and Irish were the original settlers on the land offered by William Penn. Deeply religious, frugal, and hardworking, they have passed on these values through the generations.

How could Lancastrians be expected to react to advocacy proposals? They would look carefully at any proposed expenditure for a new service, but would be ready also to act on their deeply held concern for people. Similarly, they could be expected to support advocacy that insists on systems functioning for people rather than against them.

Turning to the agency, Family and Children's Service of Lancaster County is a private family service agency staffed by fifteen professional master's degree social workers and five clerical workers. In addition to the executive director, the director of professional services oversees programs. Each program is supervised by a coordinator who also works in the program. (For example, the advocacy coordinator supervises staff advocates and works as a staff advocate herself on many issues.) These coordinators also supervise several counselors. All meet with the director of professional services to coordinate program planning and staffing.

The agency's major funding source is the United Way from whom it gets the second highest allocation of the 44 agencies it funds. The agency has a solid reputation for counseling and adoption, and its proud history goes back to its founding as the Lancaster Charity Society in 1904. The agency had, as early as 1915, set up a number of agencies such as Visiting Nurse Association and the Lancaster Day Nursery and had been concerned with the need for better housing, care of dependent and neglected children and a probation office. Gradually by the forties and fifties, however, this community emphasis had declined and had been taken over by the Lancaster Community Council. Prior to 1973 when Allen Smith arrived as a new director and the agency began thinking about setting up an advocacy program, social action at Family and Children's Service had been largely limited to the Public Issues Committee which occasionally took positions on legislative issues.

The Board was prestigious and conscientious but separated

from the professional caseworkers whose work they scarcely understood. Likewise, caseworkers, who, prior to Smith's arrival, had not been allowed to attend board meetings except for the occasional disguised case presentations, scarcely knew the Board. It was a board and agency that fitted well into the clinical emphasis of the fifties and sixties, and that in 1974 retained its prestige as a counseling and adoption agency.

The staff had not been involved in the Public Issues Committee or in social action prior to this; they were highly trained, professional caseworkers whose major involvement and identity was with clinical counseling. For the new executive to ask them to become generic caseworkers who would advocate and do family life education was a major shift from the past.

Advocacy was seen as an opportunity to return to the concern for social action that had been a proud contribution of the agency historically; the agency could now respond to the challenge of the seventies to deal with cause issues through an advocacy program, not merely on a case-by-case basis. Advocacy provided an opportunity for total agency involvement in a program; board members could work in partnership with staff members and other community people to resolve cause issues. In addition, through working together, the board and staff would come to an enriched understanding of their functions in the various programs of the agency.

An additional concern, as the Committee began to think through the program, was whether the United Way of Lancaster County would support or reject an advocacy program. A short time earlier they had developed a position on controversial issues out of concern for the backlash in allegedly reduced United Way giving following a member agency's stance (the YWCA) in favor of gun control. The United Way's position was supportive of social action; it recognized "the obligation, right and responsibility of member agencies to become involved in social issues through social action and advocacy efforts when that involvement may contribute to the elimination of community problems. At the same time, it recognizes that a member agency's public statements through the mass media may be prejudicial to the fund raising efforts" (1974) and thus adversely affect funding for programs of other agencies.

It held the board of each member agency responsible for public pronouncements, and asked that the latter be restricted to those areas where "the agency has recognized competence and knowledge". It asked further that the agency inform the United Way prior to taking a controversial stand, and held out the possibility of a conference to explore the effect on the United Way and its affiliated agencies. Finally, the United Way reserved the right to remove the agency from funding membership if it found that an agency's position was prejudicial to the

37

family of United Way agencies. The message was one of support for advocacy within certain constraints. Since the United Way is the agency's major funding source, it could do well to listen. The Board's response to the United Way's position was to insist on remaining autonomous regarding controversial issues, but to agree to alert them if the agency were getting into a controversial area.

It is important to note here that community advocacy involves both respect for the community and respect for one's autonomy and mission as an agency. Advocating about community issues and systems means that one must recognize that one continues to live in and depend on the community; advocates cannot come in and stir up the community, and then leave. They must stay to continue the agency's mission, often in ways other than advocacy. This is not to say that "outside" advocates who help us look at blind spots we would never see may not be useful at a given point, but agencies who have to go on with their work for years in the same community and depend on it for its support financially cannot operate that way. Perhaps it is analagous to marital counseling: there are certain limits on the therapist and on the couple in order not to undermine further what may be a faltering relationship; however, there is scope for change and growth within the relationship, if all operate with candor, tact and caring.

With advocacy defined, and community and agency constraints identified, let me move to what went into designing the advocacy program.

DESIGNING THE STRUCTURE

It was not easy to work out the structure for an advocacy program, but what made it possible were: an executive who believed in, and understood, advocacy; several excellent conceptual thinkers who had been involved in various social action efforts; a chairman who insisted on clear "flow" from issue to outcome, with staff and board understanding what we wanted to achieve. For me, advocacy released the social reformer, long bottled up in the family caseworker's commitment to self-determination of the client!

The Committee struggled with which of the suggested alternative program designs in the proposal would work for the agency. They wanted the program to move from case to cause, thus assuring that issues were based in the experience of clients. They also wanted the program to be accountable "up and down" to board and staff in order to receive their sanction and support. Since they could not afford much staff time, they hoped to augment the people power available to work on issues through use of board and community volunteers working closely with staff. They knew that, in addition to influential board members, the advocacy power base would be strengthened by allying with people who had experienced the problem about which they would advocate. In order that the program would be managed adequately, it became clear that staff direction would be needed on a day-to-day level, with a board-staff committee to oversee it to ensure that advocates were on the right track on issues. As they considered the characteristics of the Lancaster community, they thought that the program should be activist, not radical, in order to gain the respect and cooperation of the community.

The Committee developed the following design:

- Caseworkers would be asked to log issues from their caseloads, thus providing a written record of the issue for review. (See Advocacy Log form in Appendix 2.)

- A half-time staff person would direct the program.

- An Advocacy Committee, chaired by a board member, and composed of board, staff and community volunteers would meet monthly to review advocacy logs, to recommend issues for advocacy work and to provide oversight of the program.

- Issues would be chosen, based on certain criteria that were in keeping with overall agency goals and the specific objectives of the advocacy program. (See Criteria for Choosing Issues later in this chapter and Goals and Objectives in Chapter Four.)

- Committees, known as study-action teams (SAT's) would work on issues.

- Board would receive reports and recommendations from the Advocacy Committee and give final sanction to study and act on issues.

- Reports on work on given issues, after the study and action had been completed, would then become the basis for an annual report on the program and would further ensure accountability.

The flow chart in Figure 1 shows how advocacy issues begin in the case situation and move through a review process culminating in board sanction or rejection. This process and the rationale behind it will be described now with the use of a case situation logged by one of our counseling supervisors.

The advocacy process begins with the staff member logging the advocacy issue. (See log form in Appendix 2.) The following log is reduced for our purposes here.

FLOW CHART FOR ADVOCACY ISSUES

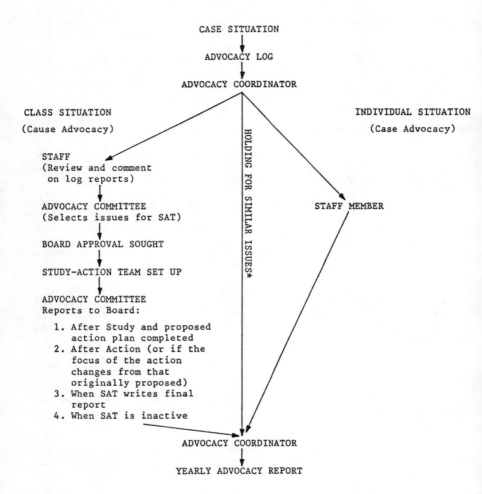

CASE SITUATION

ADVOCACY LOG

ADVOCACY COORDINATOR

CLASS SITUATION
(Cause Advocacy)

INDIVIDUAL SITUATION
(Case Advocacy)

HOLDING FOR SIMILAR ISSUES*

STAFF
(Review and comment
on log reports)

ADVOCACY COMMITTEE
(Selects issues for SAT)

STAFF MEMBER

BOARD APPROVAL SOUGHT

STUDY-ACTION TEAM SET UP

ADVOCACY COMMITTEE
Reports to Board:

1. After Study and proposed
   action plan completed
2. After Action (or if the
   focus of the action
   changes from that
   originally proposed)
3. When SAT writes final
   report
4. When SAT is inactive

ADVOCACY COORDINATOR

YEARLY ADVOCACY REPORT

*These may later go to the Advocacy Committee for consideration
when it is clear that the issue affects many families.

This chart illustrates the advocacy process: how issues "flow"
from a case situation to board approval of a study-action team.

FIGURE 1

40

```
System Dysfunction:  Public Assistance    Log No. 25PA
                     Legal Services        Logged by: EM
                                           Date: 12/09/74

Unmet Need:  Emergency shelter

Case Situation:  Wife with four small children, bad
marriage, abusive husband, wants to leave but she says
she cannot because there is no place to go with four
small children.  Public Assistance, Court order for
support not available until she has left.

Caseworker's Actions Taken:  Counseling around
problems--no other resources offered.  This was my
response but is not the answer to her actual request,
which was for help to move out.

Obstacles to Solution of Client's Problem:  No protective
service for wives.  Assumption of law that wife remain
with husband as long as he supports.
```

Note that the log illustrates several key ingredients of
advocacy: frustration at a case level; the staff member's
inability to deal with the client's request, which is a basic
survival problem; acute awareness of the cause issue: "No
protective service for abused wives." (a gap in service) and no
Public Assistance or Court Order for support until she moves out
(dysfunctioning systems); an issue rooted in a just cause for
concern; the need for a better way to solve the problem: the
staff member suggests an emergency shelter.

The second step in the advocacy procedure is that logs are
given to the advocacy coordinator who does any necessary
preliminary work up on the viability of the issue prior to making
up a log report for the monthly Advocacy Committee meeting. In
this case, the legal situation and public assistance regulations
were checked relative to an abused wife's needing shelter and
support. The Pennsylvania Department of Public Welfare insists
that a woman leaving her husband must have an address before she
can apply for public assistance. The legal situation in
Pennsylvania is that a woman is not required to remain with an
abusive husband, nor will a potential divorce be jeopardized by
her leaving. If she leaves, she can immediately petition for
support, which might take up to six weeks to begin.

The coordinator also checks whether the issue meets the

Advocacy Program objectives (see Chapter Four) and the criteria for choosing issues to be set forth in this chapter.

Suggested advocacy action in the log report to the Advocacy Committee and the Board included:

(1) the need for education of women concerning their rights and possibilities of aid in this situation. (For example, if a woman goes to the Department of Welfare before she looks for housing, they can determine her eligibility. When she has found an address, DPA will give her financial assistance and will verify with the landlord that she will be able to pay rent.) Other suggested actions were:

(2) evaluation of the adequacy and availability of concrete and counseling services to help such women, (for example, there is a need for emergency shelter, particularly in cases of severe assault or homicidal attack), and

(3) the possibility of the Study-Action Team convening an inter-agency, interdisciplinary group to work on both the educational and evaluative tasks.

This preliminary checking on the legal context, the possible cooperation of other agencies and the thinking through of possible action is helpful when the Advocacy Committee meets monthly to decide on issues. This is always a matter of balance; if too much preliminary work or thinking through of an issue is done, this can reduce the excitement and investment of the Study-Action Team. Documentation of the problem is important but on this issue the assumption was that not only our own but other agencies in the community had many cases of wife abuse.

The Advocacy Committee chooses issues based on certain criteria consonant with the overall goals of the agency and the specific objectives of the Advocacy Program. These goals and objectives will be spelled out in Chapter Four. For now, look at these criteria for choosing issues and note how the issue of a shelter for abused women fits in.

Criteria for Choosing Issues

General Criteria

Is the issue appropriate to the goals of the committee and the agency?

Can this issue be handled more appropriately and capably by another agency?

Are the necessary resources and competence available to

complete the task?

Can the task be done?

What vehicle can best accomplish this task? (SAT, Coalition, letter, etc.)

Criteria for Establishing Priorities

Family-Based

Which issue or problem is hurting families most severely?

How many families are affected by this issue or problem?

Is good case-related documentation available from our agency and other sources?

Community-Based

What critical issue is receiving the least amount of attention in the community?

Motivation

Are the board and staff excited about this issue?

Will this issue elicit community involvement?

Does this issue have a good power base (actual or potential) among the people experiencing the problem?

Impact

What issue has the promise of responding the most to the least amount of strategic intervention?

Risk

Does the risk for clients, board, staff, agency and community outweigh the potential benefits?

Will this issue violate our agreement or jeopardize our relationship with United Way?

What are the risks to families and the community if we do nothing?

Note that these criteria are seen by the Advocacy Committee as useful when discussing the viability of an issue rather than as strict guidelines. The criteria were not numbered because it was felt all should be considered, and not in any order of importance.

Regarding the issue on problems of abused women, the
Advocacy Committee readily agreed to ask the Board to set up a
study-action team (SAT) to study the issue and, if appropriate,
involve community agencies and other caregivers in thinking
through the best answer in our community. This is the initial
charge to the SAT -- the limits within which the SAT will work.

("Study-Action Team" was a term deliberately chosen to
connote the total process of successful advocacy: first, study:
to know the facts behind the issue; second, action: to indicate
advocacy does not stop at study! Action includes thinking
through alternative strategies, deciding on an action plan and
implementing that plan. Study-action teams are made up of at
least one board member, one staff member as staff advocate, and
one community member, all of whom have shown an interest in the
issue. If possible, at least one or more persons who has known
the problem is invited to join. Other staff, board or community
people are brought on to the SAT as needed, either because of the
size of the work involved, their expertise or their interest in
the issue, or because they have experienced the problem. The
usual size of an SAT is from six to ten people.

The Advocacy Committee requests an initial report of the
SAT's work after three months. This report may be given verbally
but a written report is preferable using the worksheets for study
and planning for action (Appendix 7 and 8). It is usually
possible for the SAT to report: 1) any changes to the charge
within which they will work, 2) a clear statement of the problem,
3) tentative goals and objectives which might include estimates
of numbers to be served and time frames within which the
objectives might be carried out, and 4) obstacles that the SAT is
encountering.)

The Board approved setting up an SAT to study how best to help
abused women.

Study Phase

The Study-Action Team on Abused Women was composed of a
lawyer (board member), a Human Relations Committee field worker
(community member), a staff caseworker, and me, in the role of
staff advocate. The Study-Action Team began meeting in March and
April of 1975 to think through the issue and its problems and
potential for solution. The SAT decided to limit the issue to
physically abused women. Problems were encountered in
documentation since neither police, courts nor social agencies
keep statistics on abused women; abuse is "hidden" under assault
or marital conflict. In addition, the SAT learned how time
consuming and difficult the legal apparatus was for a woman

seeking support. Information on actual shelters in England and Toronto was valuable in giving ideas on how to deal with the problem. It was obvious that the SAT would need to gain community support.

Accordingly, <u>the SAT reported to the Advocacy Committee and the Board requesting support of the action plan,</u> which was to convene a meeting of community people concerned about the problem of abused women and to share the SAT's findings. (Note that the Advocacy Program's procedure insists that the SAT report back to the Board prior to taking action or if there has been a change of focus in the study. This not only keeps the Advocacy Committee and the Board fully informed but, more importantly, gains the support and prestige of the Board in potential action.)

ACTION PHASE

To pave the way for the community meeting, a letter was sent to all the community caregivers to introduce them to the concern about the situation of abused women and the findings of the SAT. The major findings were: lack of adequate services for abused women, difficulties in getting emergency public assistance and shelter, reluctance of police to go out when there are repeated calls concerning abuse, reluctance of wives to press charges against their husbands, and the cumbersome and slow legal machinery if the wife leaves.

The idea of a shelter was suggested as a respite for the woman until she decides what she wants. The advantages of a shelter were seen as a place of safety for the woman, a cooling off period for both partners, and a support in her decision-making. The man would not have to be jailed; both could be offered counseling to deal with the problems they are experiencing, and could work on their marriage if they wished.

The community caregivers were asked to come to the meeting to share their experiences with abused women and to think through the feasibility of such a shelter in Lancaster. They were also asked to bring statistics (actual or an estimate) to document the number of abused women they saw. The 24 caregivers who came to the first community meeting on May 13 included representatives from all the social agencies plus Women's Center, Planned Parenthood, YWCA, two District Justices, police, religious organizations, lawyers, Crisis Intervention, Contact, Council on Alcoholism, the Human Relations Committee, the State Health Center, Lancaster Information Center (a coordinating information and referral agency), a hospital emergency room physician and a newspaper reporter.

At the meeting the large group was divided into four small groups with two tasks. The first task was for each person to take the role of the abused wife with three small children, no

45

money and no friends, and no place to go. Obviously, this was to involve the group in empathizing with the problem faced by abused women. These reactions were noted silently on paper by each group member and then each small group shared their findings and set up priorities for what they thought were the most urgent problems.

The second task was for the professional to take his/her own role and to list the problems he/she faced in helping the abused woman. After doing this individually, the findings were again shared in the small group and then the total findings were brought back to the large group who set final priorities on the problems faced by professionals who wanted to help abused women. Significantly, the most pressing problem felt by the professionals was their own helplessness in assisting women. No doubt this was a major reason why, when the chairperson asked who would like to work on these problems, the answer was, "Invite us all back!"

Two weeks later, the community group returned full force to look at the problems they had listed in the previous meeting. The problem areas were: helplessness of the helping person, lack of resources to deal with the problem, lack of an identifiable coordinator of service to call for help, a need for housing on a temporary basis, income maintenance for food, clothing, and shelter, counseling to support the person in the immediate crisis and help to think through problems after the emergency is past. Other problem areas noted were: ignorance of legal rights, societal attitudes such as "women's place is in the home", psychological problems of husband and wife, and the cumbersome legal machinery.

Documentation of abuse by those agencies and professionals in the group was estimated at 700 abused women per year in a county population of 361,000. Overlapping of reporting was recognized but thought to be inconsequential in view of the lack of statistics on abuse from the Police Department, Crisis Intervention, and the Council on Alcoholism.

A Shelter for Abused Women plus a coordinating counselor, knowledgeable about community resources and the problems faced by the abused woman were seen as a more complete answer to the problems faced by both abused women and professionals. A shelter would provide protection and a warm, supportive environment. The community group saw the woman as very vulnerable after the crisis of abuse and in need of help to think through the next steps. As she felt stronger, through the counseling of the shelter's staff and the support of other women in the shelter, she would be more able to move out on her own or re-establish her marriage. Thirty days in the shelter was thought to be a reasonable time.

The shelter was seen as a more viable answer for all

agencies to use as a resource when dealing with abused wives. It would be an alternative for police instead of arresting husbands, and it would provide an address for the woman to be eligible for Public Assistance and support from her husband.

A small group representing community agencies was chosen to write a proposal on how the problem could be handled. (Note that SAT members were included in the group of people from key agencies who wrote the first proposal but they continued to function now on behalf of the community.)

The community group voted to become the Lancaster Action Coalition for Abused Women on July 3 and approved a proposal to use the second floor of the YWCA residence to shelter up to twelve women and children. The plan was for a project director and five counselors who would be on rotating shifts to provide daily 24-hour coverage. This proposal was submitted to the Governor's Justice Commission on July 8 to seek funds for the shelter. Funding was denied, most Commission members feeling that a shelter was not crime prevention but social service.

I had served as the chairperson for the community meetings until the Fall of 1975. At that time the Coalition elected a district justice as its chairperson; in addition, four hard-working committees were organized: a Steering Committee, a Fact-Finding Committee, an Education/Publicity/Recruitment Committee, and a Funding Committee. The agency's executive director, who had been active in the community meetings, assumed a major role on the Funding Committee. Former members of the SAT volunteered for committees and remained active in the Coalition, and by October the Coalition for Abused Women was a vital entity in its own right. The agency's Advocacy Committee and the Board were advised that a coalition had been formed. The agency's advocacy effort had been spun off to become a community responsibility.

Efforts to get Mental Health/Mental Retardation to fund the shelter met with interest but no dollars. Publicity in newspapers and a presentation to United Way were calculated to arouse concern and possible future funding. In May of 1976, the Community Action Program (CAP) proposal writer, who served on the Coalition's Funding Committee, became aware of a potential grant to his agency. The local CAP Board enthusiastically chose the Shelter proposal over other items needing funding, and the Shelter for Abused Women began in the YWCA Residence on August 15, 1976. It was the third shelter in Pennsylvania.

The Shelter, now called Women Against Abuse, has been extremely busy ever since, often having a waiting list. Over 250 women and more than 500 children are cared for in a given year. Because of the demand the Shelter Advisory Committee looked for its own building and moved into it two years later.

The review of advocacy issues from the time they are logged, taken to the Advocacy Committee and reach the Board for final approval acts as a clarifying and creative process. The study-action team further enlarges and refines the facts behind the issue and works out the most appropriate and strategic action plan. This process, in the particular issue of abused women, provided the launching pad for an extremely effective and committed coalition.

I hope that the work toward the Shelter for Abused Women has given you some idea of how one agency's advocacy structure works and how advocating for a cause proceeds.

Let us assume that you have designed your own workable structure and are at the point of selecting advocates for your program committee or your committees to work on issues. Where can you get advocates and how will you choose those that will be most able?

RECRUITMENT, SELECTION AND TRAINING OF ADVOCATES

Since you will need to recruit advocates from staff, board and the community, begin by asking for volunteers from staff and board, then choose community professionals or other community volunteers who are concerned and knowledgeable about the issue to advocate with you. People who are experiencing the problem can be your greatest source of power and knowledge about the issue. Ask them to ally themselves with you to work on the problems.

Staff and board involvement in an advocacy program can be enhanced by expecting advocacy work as part of their job. However, it is important to give staff and board members the freedom to choose the issues on which they wish to advocate. One must be concerned in order to advocate successfully on an issue. The agency should set forth expectations of advocacy work in a caseworker's job description and in criteria for evaluation. Remember, too, that staff need to receive credit in their statistics for the time spent in advocacy work.

To enhance your advocacy program in the long term, choose staff with advocacy skills when hiring, and elect people with advocacy skills to the board, just as you would people with skills in finance and public relations.

Often, as the staff advocate, you will need to choose whom to ask to work with you. Selection of who would make a good advocate can be based on a number of criteria. You could base your choice initially on the person's previous training, volunteer or life experience. For example, you will find volunteers who have had experience in the League of Women Voters or other advocate organizations, previous training as a community organizer, lobbyist or attorney, and/or life experience that has included actual experience or awareness of the problem about which you are advocating. In addition, the following qualities are essential: the ability to think through an issue, the ability to stay with a difficult problem, the ability to work with others, and the ability to be productively assertive and comfortable about being an activist. Avoid choosing people who talk assertively but who become passive and tongue-tied when their assertiveness is needed in dialogue with an offending system or to defend a proposal for a new service.

Training of advocates is essential to help them feel ready to tackle the advocacy work. Try to provide training for total staff and board members as well as your community volunteers. You will need to do this at regular intervals of every two to three years since board and community volunteers as well as some staff will be changing.

Training for advocacy can be obtained from workshops organized by the social work profession or through long or short-term courses in Schools of Social Work. (Consult the Council on Social Work Education). The Family Advocacy Network was organized by advocates working in family service agencies to provide support and training in advocacy work to one another. The Network is not active in all parts of the country, but where it is, regular workshops are held, usually semi-annually. Invite knowledgeable advocates to your community to provide a workshop for advocates or individual agency consultation. Consult your professional accrediting body for names of appropriate consultants or training opportunities. Build a library. Train yourself and then train others.

Let us move now to how you can orient and empower your total staff and board to advocate, or at a minimum, to understand their role in supporting the advocacy program.

REFERENCES

MANSER, E. (ed.) (1973) Family Advocacy: A Manual for Action. New York: Family Service Association of America.

FOUR

ORIENTATION AND EMPOWERMENT

Now that you have designed your advocacy program and have chosen advocates to work on issues, how will you bring the rest of your board and staff to the point of awareness that you and those who worked to set up your program have? Your board and staff will need to be oriented to what advocacy is and how it will work in your agency; they, too, need to feel empowered to advocate successfully.

Some ways to do this are: circulation of a memo, orientation at a staff meeting and at a board meeting, orientation at a workshop for board and staff, or the use of a consultant. A consultant is the easiest, if you have the funds and can find someone; if you do use a consultant, make sure that he/she involves board and staff in workshop exercises. Much better, to my mind, is an orientation workshop planned and led by your own committee who designed your program. Working together to plan what the others need to learn will also cement relationships between board and staff and will develop greater ownership of the program. The workshop would provide an opportunity, also, for your executive to come out firmly in favor of advocacy as well as to give "permission" to board and staff to take time to become used to this new way of thinking and working.

Such a workshop ought to include at least these three areas: 1) what advocacy is and how it has worked elsewhere: 2) how advocacy will work in your agency; and 3) how to become empowered to advocate.

WHAT ADVOCACY IS

A good way to decide what will be good learning for a group is to ask what helped you. You could put your board and staff through a similar process of defining advocacy for themselves to the one you went through as a committee. You could provide some key definitions (see Chapter Three), divide the large group into small groups and ask them to come up with their own definition. This is not only a good teaching technique, it is also fun.

To help your agency staff and board "see" why advocacy is needed as an important service to families, present examples of how advocacy has worked elsewhere.

HOW ADVOCACY WILL WORK IN YOUR AGENCY

The way advocacy will work in your agency will, of course, depend on your design. However a program is designed, staff will have their particular needs for orientation and empowerment and board will, too. If you orient both groups together, they will provide support and insights to one another, and begin to develop a feeling of partnership in learning together, which is an excellent preface to working together on issues.

Let me describe some of the key areas that staff and board need to understand at the outset, basically the goals upon which the advocacy program rests and the roles each would play in the advocacy process and procedures. Some of what follows will be unique to this program model, but most will be aspects that you will need to consider in your agency. Note also that some of this would be important to include in an orientation workshop, while other aspects are included to illustrate how one advocacy program works.

THE BASIS OF AN ADVOCACY PROGRAM: GOALS AND OBJECTIVES

Any program must define its purpose and how it will carry this out. As you begin, this may be relatively simple: a definition of what advocacy is for your organization and the criteria for issues that you will undertake. Obviously, these must be consonant with the purpose of your agency. If your agency has (or undertakes) a planning process that defines its goals and objectives, each program will relate to these goals in specific ways. The goals and objectives of an advocacy program can be developed more definitively as your program grows and you see the need to have basic parameters within which to work. These can form the basis from which you will evaluate your work on an annual basis. (See Chapter Eight.)

Let us look at one family service agency's overall goals and how one of these (goal c.) becomes the basis for the agency's advocacy goals. These in turn become the basis for the advocacy program goal, which become the basis for the advocacy program objectives. The following goals and objectives are taken from Lancaster County Family and Children's Service, Pa.

GOALS AND OBJECTIVES OF ONE FAMILY SERVICE AGENCY

The purpose of this non-profit corporation originally chartered for administering charity, is to facilitate the optimum development of families and individuals by providing relevant services which:

a. assist people with problems of an individual and/or interpersonal nature to either overcome such problems and/or achieve an improved level of coping with them.

b. assist people whose family or individual functioning is not impaired to build awareness and skills needed to prevent diminished functioning and/or achieve enhanced functioning;

c. attain an environment of community conditions, structures, and systems which is supportive of family and individual development.

Section c. (above) provides the broad basis for advocacy, which again is more narrowly defined in the agency's goal statement related to advocacy.

1. Develop broader community sensitivity to, and awareness of, the needs and rights of its families and individuals.

2. Actively work toward an increasingly efficient and effective matching of family and individual needs and rights to available community resources.

3. Support families or individuals to use available community resources effectively.

4. Increase the capabilities of community resources, existing and potential, to meet family and individual needs and rights.

The overall Advocacy Program goal is: to fulfill human potential by improving life conditions and insuring that community institutions work for people rather than against them.

The following Advocacy Program objectives carry out the Advocacy Program goal and the agency's goal.

1. Identify areas, through casework and other means, where needs and rights of families and individuals do not appear to be adequately served or are unmet.

2. Change systems and institutions that do not adequately serve families and individuals.

3. Create systems and institutions to serve unmet needs of families and individuals.

4. Educate individuals within systems and institutions

52

to the needs and rights of families and individuals.

5. Match the needs and rights of families and individuals with existing systems, institutions and resources.

6. Involve those people who are experiencing problems in the advocacy process whenever possible.

7. Evaluate and improve the quality of the advocacy process and the overall program on an ongoing basis.

These goals and objectives form the parameters within which staff, board and community volunteers can do the advocacy work. As I have indicated, you may be able to begin designing your program with established agency goals in mind, or you may need to develop these advocacy goals and objectives as your program develops in order to be able to evaluate what you are doing in terms of the goals and objectives set earlier. We will discuss this in greater detail in Chapter Eight.

ADVOCACY PROGRAM PROCEDURES

It is obviously vital that all staff and board understand how advocacy program procedures will be carried out as you move from case to cause--from the advocacy log to the final report of a study-action team. Make a chart of the Flow of Issues as shown in Figure 1 in Chapter Three or a similar chart of your own design and take the board and staff through the various steps that an issue will need to take. Point out the importance of their roles at each step. To clarify this, let us look at the ways staff and board members will be involved in advocacy work.

STAFF INVOLVEMENT

I will begin with the role of the executive director, move to the advocacy coordinator, and finally discuss how staff on the front line can be involved in advocacy.

ROLE OF THE EXECUTIVE DIRECTOR

The executive director is the leader in the agency. He or she sets the tone, whether of innovation and change, or maintenance of stability; he/she leads, integrates and sustains, all of which are vital in establishing and continuing an advocacy program.

An executive might foster innovation by initiating a

planning process that forces board and staff to look afresh at
what a family service agency, for example, should be doing to
meet the needs of families. Such a planning process might
include the need for advocacy as a means to work on cause issues
faced by families. A planning process is a good means of
initiating discussion about advocacy or other new programs
because it involves the total agency (board and staff) and
usually looks for evaluative community input. Planning involves
the kind of discussion, thinking through and voting on priorities
that helps to integrate the new with the more familiar agency
functions.

The executive shows his/her leadership by allocation of
staff time to work in the program, also by allocation of board
time to learn about the program and sanction its activities. In
addition, he/she is the one to encourage broad staff and board
participation on study-action teams. By his/her stance as a
proponent of advocacy for the agency, and working as an advocate
in certain key situations, the executive manifests a commitment
to the value of the advocacy program, thus sustaining and
supporting it.

ROLE OF THE ADVOCACY COORDINATOR

When deciding on staff for this role, look for someone with
a deep commitment to the professional and ethical base on which
advocacy rests, and with a clear conviction about the right to
advocate. In addition, the person who leads the agency in
advocacy awareness and effort must have the freedom to risk, the
courage to face difficult situations and the patience to
persevere when the going is long, and possibly rough. Overall,
the advocate and/or coordinator must have management skills and
be able to work well with people in the program. He/she must
have the capacity to empower the task group, encourage and
support its efforts, and appreciate its achievements.

The specific roles and responsibilities of the advocacy
coordinator include:

Leadership to staff and board in the initial planning and
ongoing refining of the advocacy program; to the Advocacy
Committee and its chairperson regarding both the overall program
and the details of process in a given SAT, for example. The
coordinator advocates for advocacy as a method of helping people,
and promotes integration of advocacy work into overall agency
goals and programs. The coordinator takes a leadership role in
raising the consciousness of the staff regarding advocacy
issues—both case and cause advocacy—in their caseloads and
raising the consciousness of board regarding advocacy issues in
the community.

Empowerment through infusing all of the participants in an

54

advocacy program, lay and professional, paid and volunteer, with a sense of the power they bring to advocacy work, their particular talents and strengths, their insights and ideas, their expertise and value as persons.

Supervision of the advocacy process through consultation with staff advocates regarding their work on SATs and coalitions.

Orientation of all board and staff to what advocacy is and how it is carried out in the agency. (See Figure 1 in Chapter Three and Figures 2-6 in Chapter 6.)

Disposition of logs in the light of agency goals and advocacy program objectives as well as the criteria for issue selection. A decision must be made whether a given log should be worked on as a case advocacy issue by the caseworker or whether there is sufficient basis to send the log on as a cause issue to the Advocacy Committee for their review and disposition. In certain issues the log will be held pending receipt of more logs on that issue or greater evidence of documentation of the problem. (See Figure 1 in Chapter Three.)

Record keeping. The original logs are filed by number and cross-referenced when there are multi-system problems so that it is easy to assess in annual reports the systems in which problems are appearing. Log files and all advocacy reports become the ongoing records of the program.

Compilation of educational and program resources.

Consultation with legal resources to clarify the legal implications and context of an advocacy issue. The agency's legal consultant or the local Legal Services' staff can be consulted regarding low-income families.

Management of the total program in order that all aspects function as smoothly as possible. It is, of course, necessary to work closely with the executive director, the director of professional services, and coordinators of other agency programs such as counseling, adoption, and family life education, to keep them aware of the need for staff time and the scope of advocacy efforts. This is necessary particularly when planning allocation of staff to each agency program.

EXPECTATIONS OF STAFF

For staff an advocacy program is both a resource and a responsibility: a resource through which their clients' system problems can be dealt with, a responsibility to log issues seen in their casework or family life education experience. One way to encourage this is to make advocacy awareness and involvement part of each worker's evaluation. All caseworkers can be expected to log issues that they see in their work with families; however, participation in advocacy study-action work may be voluntary. The message from administration and board can be that advocacy awareness is a requirement for today's social worker. "Front line" caseworkers in a family service (or other human service) agency are in a unique position to hear and report the systemic problems that their clients face. This knowledge can become the documentation for a vital advocacy effort.

Obstacles to Awareness:

Even when the expectations of administration are clear, a number of obstacles can hinder the awareness of a need for advocacy. For example, the caseworker could be struggling with whether a situation is really the "fault" of the client or whether the client could, in fact, be somewhat paranoid: that is, he/she might be looking at the intrapsychic and inter-relationship factors without clearly "hearing" the system problems and diagnosing those. The caseworker needs to risk believing the client's view. The beginning of advocacy diagnosis is committing to the client rather than the system. For years caseworkers have had little choice but to help clients "adjust" to faulty systems or to try to work out amelioration on a one-to-one basis as in case advocacy. This has led to a discounting of the client's problem with a bureaucracy. Sunley, (1970), in his discussion of the caseworker's feelings, points out that because the client might not have "clean hands", the worker might not see that the client's legal or human rights have been violated; or he/she could be a person who identifies strongly with authority and could rationalize that although authorities make mistakes, they mean well. There might also be a tendency to think: "Some other agency (perhaps the local legal services) can do it better; our job is casework."

It is true also that the term advocacy sometimes seems like "agitating" and confrontation is uncomfortable for some caseworkers. However, caseworkers will feel better when they realize that just as confrontation is necessary for growth in an individual or family therapy situation, it is vital that systems be confronted in order that they do not continue to work against the very people they were set up to help.

Enabling Factors

Commitment to advocacy as a method of helping comes when caseworkers see the Advocacy Program as a resource just as they would see any other community resource. Caseworkers have always done case advocacy; they need to go a step farther into cause advocacy. Caseworkers need to feel that there is a payoff for them and their clients in alerting the advocacy program to potential issues. The payoff for the caseworker comes in terms of helping clients deal with more of their problems and helping them assert their rights. They can feel also that they are helping many people not known to them.

The payoff for clients is, first, in being heard, in knowing that the caseworker cares; second, in feeling that something can be done about their frustration with a system; and, third, in their possibly being involved in study-action teams to try to solve the problem. They might also become part of a group of clients and others who are empowered to do their own advocating. To become involved in an advocacy effort will provide constructive use of their anger; success will produce growth and strengthened egos. Advocacy thus becomes a treatment resource as well.

You will need to address these issues in staff meetings as well as in joint board and staff orientation sessions. The following guides can help staff to begin logging issues. (See Advocacy Log form in Appendix 2.)

The Purpose of Logging Advocacy Issues

1. To provide a means to identify cause issues, classes of problems/issues/ obstacles that are affecting many people, not just one client.

2. to identify specific problems in which systems are functioning against people rather than for them.

3. To identify gaps in service within or between agencies, where clients are "falling between the cracks". Note especially intake requests that cannot be met.

4. To provide an opportunity to look at the agency's own system (internal advocacy). Log any practice or policy pursued that you feel has a negative impact on clients.

5. To identify problems that may be common to clients in other agencies also. This could lead to inter-agency or other group coalitions.

6. To provide a basis for seeing over the course of a year's work what advocacy issues were present in the agency's caseload. An annual report on the Advocacy Program will incorporate these findings.

How to Spot an Advocacy Issue

1. Individual situation - client powerless: Is it a situation in which your client cannot deal with the system to get what he or she is entitled to receive? This could mean the "right" morally to be treated as a human being, or the "right" legally, according to existing regulations in the system.

2. Cause or class situation - many people powerless: Is it a situation in which many families or individuals known to you or your client cannot deal with the system to obtain their rights?

3. Caseworker powerless: Is it a situation in which you as a caseworker cannot deal with the system to obtain what you see clients should be entitled to?

4. System dysfunctional: Is the system working against your clients rather than for them? Note where the dysfunction is in the system.

5. Unmet needs: Are there gaps in service?

6. Unmet rights: Are there general human rights or specific groups (e.g. women, poor or others) that are not provided for or protected?

Log all situations in which you have seen a need for advocacy (externally or internally), whether you have done anything about it or not. Of course, if you have dealt with the situation, indicate what you have done.

(See exercise at the end of this chapter for a means to help staff and others identify cause issues from a case situation.)

You may wish to limit logging of issues to staff initially so as not to be overwhelmed. Later, board members could be invited to log issues that they see, which are of community concern. This will involve them in the program as well as broaden the base from which issues come.

In addition to logging issues, staff need to understand the various ways they might participate in advocacy. For instance, they may volunteer to work on SAT's, represent staff on the Advocacy Committee, and review all log reports prior to referral to the Advocacy Committee. The latter is important to keep staff abreast of issues that are being identified as well as to offer an opportunity to share their ideas regarding possible solutions or additional documentation of the problem. The major staff involvement as staff advocate on an SAT will be discussed in Chapter Five.

BOARD INVOLVEMENT

Let us move now from staff involvement in the advocacy program to how board members can fulfill vital roles there also.

58

Role of the Board

Commitment of the Board to the idea of advocacy is of primary importance both to the initial setting up of the program and to its continued success. This does not mean that every board member has to be convinced, but a majority must be ready to commit themselves to the agency's purpose of fostering systems that work for people rather than against them. The Board's commitment forms the ideological basis for sanction of the program. Commitment to advocacy as an idea and as a program prompts the Board to defend the allocation of staff time to advocacy during budget review by funding bodies.

The Board can carry out its commitment to advocacy through two vital roles: first, <u>sanction</u> of the overall program, as well as sanction to set up individual study-action teams to work on particular cause issues; and second, <u>participation</u> of individual board members in the advocacy work of the Advocacy Committee and/or on SAT's.

Without the Board's sanction, advocacy would be very weak indeed. It is the thoughtful, involved backing of representative citizens of the community working on behalf of a respected agency that gives an advocacy program its strength. This is not to deny the influence and expertise of professionals within an agency or their allies from the community, which, combined with board strength, produces significant advocate power. It does seem, however, that funding groups and community decision-makers are more easily persuaded when board members and other citizens are convinced of a need or an institutional reform. Perhaps funding sources are suspicious of professionals who advocate for a need in situations where their profession could be expected to do the job; perhaps they see social workers or other human service professionals as "do-gooders." Whatever the true case, board backing of an advocacy program, in general, and on particular issues, is imperative.

The Board carries out its role of sanction in the following ways:

1. Setting up the advocacy program, in concert with the overall goals and program planning of the agency;

2. Allocating oversight of the Advocacy Program to the Advocacy Committee, which acts as a mini-board to make sure that advocates operate within the guidelines of the program;

3. Voting on the Advocacy Committee's recommendations for means (usually SAT's) to carry out the program; and,

4. Assigning the Advocacy Committee to evaluate the efficacy of the Advocacy Program.

1. Board Sets Up the Advocacy Program

The Board's role in setting up the program was described in Chapter One where the Board set up the ad hoc Committee to Study the Feasibility of a Family Advocacy Program. The Committee's first report recommended advocacy as an integral part of the agency's programs, defined advocacy, and suggested a pilot program to work out how to process issues and work on them.

2. Board Allocates Oversight to the Advocacy Committee

The Board allocates oversight of the operation of the Advocacy Program to the Advocacy Committee and is closely involved by virtue of the fact that five board members serve on the committee, one of whom is the chairperson. In addition, four community members (volunteers chosen by board or staff members), two staff caseworkers, the advocacy coordinator and the executive director, who are both advisory, make up the committee. The Advocacy Committee chairperson works closely with the advocacy coordinator in matters of program and process. The chairperson's role is described later in this chapter.

The Responsibilities of the Advocacy Committee

--to ensure that the Advocacy Program is operating within the overall agency goals and objectives and its own specific goals and objectives. Thus, each issue brought to the Advocacy Committee must be looked at in terms of whether working on that issue will further the goals and objectives of the Advocacy Program.

--to ensure that the procedures for the flow of issues from staff to board as outlined in Figure 1 are followed.

--to decide which advocacy issues documented in log reports should take priority, using the Criteria for Choosing Issues detailed in Chapter Three. Of paramount importance is the question of whether the agency has the resources and competence to complete the advocacy task. Does the agency have the people (board, staff and community) with time and expertise to work on a particular issue? If not, this might involve foregoing an otherwise viable issue. It is easy, given the power of issues to move people to action, to think that they can do more than can be expected with their time and energy. Advocacy committees and coordinators have to be careful to avoid burnout among staff and volunteers.

Let me interrupt our thinking about the responsibilities of the Advocacy Committee to talk about the kind of issues that an agency takes on. Perhaps you would like to hear of some examples. Here are some typical issues:

--advocating that a school district fund a learning center that had been recommended by its faculty but vetoed by the superintendent year after year.

--developing a Bereaved Parents Support Group and educating professionals in grief counseling.

--beginning a program of Friendly Visitors to Nursing Homes.

--working in various systems (legal, education, the church, counseling agencies, the state legislature) to raise their consciousness and improve services or laws for children of divorce and their parents.

--developing a Hospice.

--promoting the doctor-patient partnership by promoting a pamphlet put out in cooperation with the local Medical Society.

--through the same pamphlet and a special listing in the phone book, enabling better awareness and access to the Medical Society regarding patient grievances.

--developing lesson plans for teachers to discuss stress and suicide prevention with adolescents and where to turn for help.

--developing in-agency custody mediation services and a divorce mediation program.

--advocating that superintendents of school districts make possible better identification of learning disabled students and more in-service training for regular classroom teachers of minimally learning disabled students.

--advocating for low and moderate income housing.

--confronting dysfunctioning in the Social Security Office and the Unemployment Claims Office.

--raising the consciousness of local newspapers regarding their accounts of suicide and also of child abuse (the former causing the family additional grief, the latter so sensationalized that doctors feared parents would not bring their abused children for needed medical care.)

You will note that these issues have included new programs, new services, improvement of services in dysfunctional systems, consciousness raising and educating and lobbying the legislature regarding improved laws.

What issues might your agency take on if you had an
advocacy program?

Let us return to the remaining responsibilities of the
Advocacy Committee. They are:

--to recommend how a given issue should be handled, such as
through a study-action team, coalition or position paper.
Usually the committee recommends an SAT, as most issues require
thorough study and planning of strategy prior to action. In some
instances the committee will recommend that the agency join in a
coalition from the outset. The coalition functions similarly to
an SAT but is not under the jurisdiction of the board. However,
consistent reporting of the agency's involvement in a coalition
is relayed to the Advocacy Committee and Board. In other
instances the Advocacy Committee might feel that there is
insufficient time for board and staff to work with thoroughness
on an issue; in such situations position papers or letters from
the Board and/or executive may be used to convey the agency's
concern.

--to refine the advocacy issue chosen into a motion to Board
to set up the advocacy vehicle, usually an SAT. The wording of
the motion is important because this statement of the problem and
what the advocates want permission to do then becomes the
"charge" to the SAT regarding the problem and the limits within
which they will work.

62

--to seek volunteers to work on a particular issue;

--to monitor and offer consultation to ongoing SAT's in monthly Advocacy Committee meetings using the Guide for Evaluation of a Study-Action Team (see Figure 4 in Chapter Six) to be discussed shortly;

--to review and evaluate the initial report (after three months), interim reports (study phase, action plans) or final reports of SAT's prior to taking these to the Board for their approval;

--to appoint Advocacy Committee members to sit on community committees or review boards consonant with the agency's advocacy goals (for example, Community Development Review);

--to review the annual report of the advocacy program and evaluate the program and process. (See guide to do this and full discussion in Chapter Eight.)

3. Board Votes on the Advocacy Committee's Recommendations:

At its monthly meeting the Board hears a report from the chairperson of the Advocacy Committee regarding any of the foregoing aspects of the Committee's work. Significant aspects of the SAT's and community coalitions are shared for information. The Board approves (or rejects) requests from the committee to set up an SAT, and expects an interim report on the study and proposed action prior to the SAT's entrance into the action phase. This keeps the SAT accountable and the board informed. Note that board members will become increasingly comfortable about sanctioning advocacy work when they are kept involved and knowledgeable about each stage of advocacy efforts, so that questions from their friends and colleagues in the community about what the agency is doing do not take them by surprise.

Board approval provides the SAT the sanction necessary for strong or controversial action. During the life of an SAT any marked change in the charge from that which was originally approved must be taken back to the board.

The Board will vote also on recommended changes in advocacy program structure and/or procedures.

4. Board Receives an Evaluation of the Advocacy Program:

The Advocacy Committee appoints an ad hoc Evaluation Committee to do a yearly assessment of the efficacy of the Advocacy Program on the basis of SAT reports and the annual review of other advocacy activities. The findings of this

Evaluation Committee become part of the program's annual report, which is given to the board and staff.

5. Board Participates in the Advocacy Program:

Another role, and possibly the most interesting for the board members, is participation on the Advocacy Committee and in advocacy work on SAT's or in community coalitions. They also occasionally log issues, and represent the agency on citizen review boards that have relevance to the agency's advocacy goals. If you are a board member or an executive wondering where you will get people to work on advocacy issues, you may be encouraged by the view of a former board president who was active in the Advocacy Program. Mrs. Desch (1980) says:

> The major reward for me, as a board member is that I have a better understanding and feel more a part of the agency for the simple reason that an advocacy program is highly visible. . . . I come from volunteer work at the YWCA. There, if you want to see a program in action, go in to the gym or drop in on one of the informal education classes or the child care center, and it's all happening right before your eyes. At F&CS, in contrast, you walk down a corridor of closed doors. While I understand the reason intellectually, I don't think I every really got used to that during my six years there. Think about the volunteers on your board. Their experiences are probably similar whether they come out of YW, YM, Boy Scouts, Girl Scouts, etc. and while counseling does (and must) go on behind closed doors, an advocacy program can open those doors with the visibility it provides for the agency in the community.

Board, staff, community volunteers (professional and lay) and people with the problem work together on SAT's and coalitions. The board member's presence provides prestige; his/her ideas and analysis of the problem provide strength for the advocates' "case:" the board member's commitment as an advocate provides support to the other members of the team on the uphill road of advocacy and gives evidence of the agency's belief in the cause.

Role of the Chairperson on the Advocacy Committee:

The Advocacy Committee's chairperson is a board member. His/her role is extremely important in guiding, enabling, and suggesting improvements to program procedures. The chairperson's various tasks are:

--to chair the monthly Advocacy Committee meeting where new logs are presented and SAT's monitored. He/she makes sure as well that advocacy procedures are adhered to and takes a leadership role in suggesting modifications to structure or process that would improve performance.

--to recruit board members for the Advocacy Committee who are not only interested in and knowledgeable about advocacy but who are willing to work on SAT's or other advocacy work. Lack of attendance or participation is dealt with by the chairperson. The chairperson and the coordinator, or other members of the committee, suggest and recruit community members.

--to report to the Board, which includes getting permission to form new SAT's, reporting periodically on their progress or final reports on SAT's, sharing the annual report of the Advocacy Program, and reporting on any other areas of interest or concern to the board. He/she must have the tact and skill to deal effectively with reactions and suggestions from the Board so as to educate them in the ongoing advocacy effort, to help the board to feel involved and vital to the sanction or ending of a particular advocacy effort, and to incorporate their thinking into that which has been done previously.

--to work with and support the coordinator and other advocates in the rigors and rewards of advocacy work.

Prime requisites for the Advocacy Committee chairperson, the executive director, and the advocacy coordinator are a sense of humor and a capacity for objectivity to help fellow advocates see beyond the momentary setbacks and to look more realistically at their capacities and limitations.

We have been concerned about how you will bring your board and staff to the same point of understanding and enthusiasm that your committee designing the program has begun to feel. We need to move now from the intellectual understanding of what advocacy is and how it might work in an agency to how you will infuse your potential advocates with the feeling that they _can_ advocate.

EMPOWERMENT

In Chapter Two we talked about the right to advocate and the basis from which that is derived in a social agency. The following is an idea for a "lead in" to a discussion on empowerment in an orientation workshop for board and staff: divide the group into several small groups; their task is to write down their four worst fears about advocating and their four best hopes. This helps to deal with negative and positive feelings; these feelings can be shared later in the full group and recognized as valid. The exercise should allow the group to "hear" better the bases for the right to advocate, where power comes from, and the potency of joining together in a just cause. Refer back to Chapter Two for general areas that you will need to consider in empowering people.

I would like to add a few more specifics on empowering board members, people who are experiencing the problem, and staff.

EMPOWERING BOARD MEMBERS

It is not difficult to orient and empower most board members, particularly if you have selected those who have a commitment to advocacy. When you begin you will be fortunate if a good proportion of the board are advocacy minded. As board terms expire, it is important for a nominating committee to keep in mind the need for advocates. Just as the agency needs financial wizards, public relations experts, planners and others, the board also needs people who might have struggled with unyielding systems or are aware of gaps in community services.

Although a board needs a number of members who are advocacy minded, Desch (1980), reminds us: "Believe it or not, you need the skeptics. Since every board has at least one, make the most efficient use of that negativism . . . You can be assured that all the doubts that the board skeptic expresses will probably be raised by your staff skeptic . . . When someone asks: 'How will it work? What are the risks? Who will give that much time?' those questions force us to think through the process more clearly."

In addition to skepticism, some board members will need their consciousness raised: for example, concerning what it means to be poor and powerless, or the racist implications of decisions, not only in their own agency, but in other organizations and with other people with whom they come in contact.

Empowering board members is less difficult than empowering staff or people experiencing the problem because board members know they carry the authority for agency policy and the responsibility for appropriate agency service in the community. Many board members are community leaders and accustomed to exercising their power. They also find satisfaction in going beyond their objective roles as monitors and policy makers to actually working on cause issues that confront families.

EMPOWERING PEOPLE WHO ARE EXPERIENCING THE PROBLEM

An advocate group can become the catalyst to enable a community to face its need and join together to do something about it. As an example, agency advocates served as a catalyst by calling a meeting of community leaders to discuss the need for a teen recreation center in a nearby suburb. Caseworkers had become concerned about the lack of after-school supervision for young teens in homes where mothers and fathers worked or where mothers were the sole support. Schools referred children for counseling because of drug use and sexual promiscuity. Discussion with the parents and teens revealed that there was little constructive recreational activity for these youngsters, and they were too young to work. The YWCA and YMCA were in the city, 15 miles away, and these teens had no transportation. Children in a large rental complex were not even allowed to throw frisbees within the grounds. Contact with community leaders revealed that a number of persons had seen the need for a supervised recreation center (which was being suggested by the SAT) but no one had taken the initiative to call a meeting.

Professionals, too, can need the support and expertise of advocacy programs. A legal aid lawyer, having previously worked on the Coalition for Abused Women, called to discuss his concern about whether agencies in the community were sufficiently meeting the needs of a quadriplegic client of his. She was threatened with losing custody of her 18-month old child because she could not care for him herself after her husband left them. The agency called a conference of relevant agencies at which the lack of services for the severely handicapped and the poor coordination of those that were available became starkly evident. Several case advocacy conferences were held to try to help and plan for this client. The fact that her only alternative at age 32 was placement of her child in a foster home, and care for herself was available only in a nursing home for aged, catapulted the agency into an advocacy study-action team for adequate living arrangements for severely handicapped, mentally alert, adults. (This is, of course, an excellent example of "case to cause".)

Empowering people who have the problem might not be easy. Often, they are already overburdened with family problems (as with abused women), with poverty, or the debilitating effects of racism. Because of their multiple problems, they may have very low self esteem. They feel themselves to be the least powerful in our society. They mistrust society's institutions, believe that nothing will change, and feel varying degrees of alienation from society. (Solomon, 1976:25) She stresses the necessity of taking into account how much a group's sense of powerlessness derives "from the experience of systematic negative valuation based on membership in a stigmatized racial or ethnic group." I would add "or being poor or on welfare." Solomon cautions that "empowerment activities must be designed to insure that the problem-solving process itself serves to counteract the negative valuations." She suggests that we pay attention to different perceptions on the part of white and black clients. White clients may expect advocacy as their due. Black clients may feel "they're doing something for me because they didn't want me to do it for myself" or "because they believe I am incompetent."

Solomon offers four goals for empowering those who feel most powerless in our society. The client or other person should be helped to:

1. See himself as a change agent capable of achieving a solution to his problem. He knows the problem.

2. See the advocate as having knowledge and skills that he (the client) can use.

3. See the advocate as a partner, a person with whom he can combine forces in the problem-solving effort.

4. See the power structure as multipolar, showing varying degrees of commitment to the status quo, and therefore open to influence.

She points out that the structure of an agency program must empower. Is the service delivery system an obstacle course or an opportunity system? (Solomon, 1976:29) If empowerment of people with the problem is to succeed, advocates must be ready to join with them as allies, not as experts. The advocate-ally must see the victim as a person who may be in difficult times but communicate her/his belief that the victim is strong and capable of action. They can then work together, studying, developing strategies and acting for change. Such an alliance reduces the isolation of both the victim and the advocate, and provides the power base for action.

EMPOWERING THE STAFF

In many agencies one of the toughest tasks is to empower and involve staff in advocacy. It is not unusual to have some staff who are very committed, some lukewarm, and some who are hostile to advocacy work. Reasons for this vary from poor preparation and orientation by agency administration to poor communication about what is expected, and fear of something new and untried. In addition, caseworkers are often committed to their counseling skills and feel they do not have the time or the incentive to transfer these skills to advocacy. Many prefer the crisis work of therapy rather than work on a broad, cause issue. Many feel that they do not have the time to take on what they see as additional work.

Obviously good preparation and orientation are extremely important in empowering staff to feel that they can use their existing skills in advocacy work. They need to be reminded that diagnosing problems and coming up with solutions and interventions is what caseworkers do every day. In advocacy, the caseworker takes responsibility for organizing and enabling the advocacy group who will then work together to diagnose the problem, agree on their hoped-for solution, and think through the interventions that are possible.

Many staff members (and indeed, board or others working on an issue) will feel most highly motivated about an issue that they have logged. It is important to use that motivation if at all possible in assigning staff advocates.

Staff also need clear messages from the executive and other supervisory personnel that the work of advocacy is not "extra", but that they will be allocated time in their schedule to do it. Furthermore, they need to be aware that they will receive credit for doing advocacy from their supervisors and the executive at evaluation time and from the Board as they become aware of what the staff are doing in advocacy. Staff will need ongoing support from the advocacy coordinator and the executive. The most effective empowerment comes from success on an issue, and the recognition that comes from that internally as well as in the local community and among other professionals.

STOP AND THINK

In your agency . . .

Who could carry the role of advocacy coordinator? Advocacy Committee chairperson? Staff advocate?

What would help each of them to carry out his/her role more effectively?

Who can help to build awareness of advocacy?

Who are convinced advocates who could empower others?

How will you organize orientation of your staff and board?

What are their learning needs in relation to advocacy?

What are their empowerment needs?

Before you move to the next chapter where we will discuss the role of the staff advocate in working with the Study-Action Team, try the following exercise in choosing issues.

EXERCISE

This exercise can be used with staff, board, other professionals and volunteers to help them become aware of cause issues in a case situation. From the following case, choose: 1) all the cause issues you can; 2) the most important cause issue on which you might work. (Use the Criteria for Choosing Issues as a guide or modify those criteria to suit your organization.)

CASE SITUATION

A medical social worker from a local hospital referred Ms. Jones to Family Service. Ms. Jones is a single mother of three children, ages 10, 6 and 3. Her three-year old son is hospitalized for the third time for acute lead poisoning. The child's pediatrician refuses to discharge the child until the family finds a lead-free apartment. (There is no state or local law regarding lead paint.) The medical social worker indicated also that the 10 year old son was acting out at home and was not performing well in school.

Ms. Jones failed her first appointment at Family Service. She called the following day to reschedule. She explained that she had spent several hours at the welfare office because the worker kept her waiting two hours after her scheduled appointment.

When she came in for her second appointment, she first raised the housing issue. She had gone to the housing authority and was told there was a long waiting list. She also has spent two months looking for a new apartment, but no one wants to rent to her.

She complained that her oldest son is not minding her. She is angry that he does not come straight home from school to look after his sister while she is out looking for jobs.

REFERENCES

DESCH, S.D. and E.D. TAYLOR (1980) "Getting an Advocacy Program Started." Unpublished paper presented at Family Service Association of America Middle Atlantic Regional Council Meeting.

SOLOMON, B.B. (1976) Black Empowerment. New York: Columbia.

SUNLEY, R. (1970) "Family Advocacy: From Case to Cause." Social Casework (June) 349-350.

FIVE

THE ROLE OF THE STAFF ADVOCATE IN WORKING
WITH THE STUDY-ACTION TEAM

To help us move from structure to the actual advocacy work, let us think about the role of the staff advocate in working with the study-action team. It seems to me that there are four aspects: the staff advocate represents and carries out the agency's policy regarding advocacy, making sure that an issue proceeds through a defined process and internal structure as was discussed earlier; she/he represents and carries out the professional role of advocate using generic social work skills to problem solve and intervene effectively; she/he enables people to learn advocacy skills and empowers them to use their talents, ideas and motivation to complete the advocacy task. The staff advocate also elicits ongoing review and evaluation of the efficacy of the advocacy work. In the next two chapters we will focus on the study and action aspects of the advocacy task in which the staff advocate uses more of the agency representative and the problem-solving roles. In Chapter Eight we will look at the staff advocate's ongoing role in the annual evaluation of the advocacy work. This chapter will focus to a greater extent on his/her enabling role with the people involved in the task: how the staff advocate (along with the chairperson) can enable them to function most effectively as individuals and facilitate their process as a group to do the work.

Let us assume that you are the staff advocate organizing a new study-action team. We will consider how you will use your enabling role to organize and work with the SAT members to orient, educate and empower them. We will consider how you will evaluate the SAT's work and help the members to review their efforts. We will consider also how you will deal with some problems that are common in advocacy groups and, finally, how you will handle the ending phase of advocacy work.

ORGANIZING THE STUDY-ACTION TEAM

Your initial tasks are: deciding who should be on the SAT, inviting them, choosing a chairperson, and working with the chairperson to plan the initial meeting. You must see that orientation materials such as the advocacy log and the final charge to the SAT approved by the board are sent out to the members, along with notification of time, place and duration of the meeting. You will need to line up orientation materials for the first meeting in a study-action packet (the contents of which

71

will be discussed shortly) to guide them as they work on an issue.

CHOOSING SAT MEMBERS

An SAT should have from six to ten members, depending on the tasks ahead and the expertise needed. Larger SAT's or coalitions can be divided into sub-committees to do aspects of the work. My recommendation about the minimum composition would be one or more board members, one or more community members, and one or more persons who have experienced the problem, in addition to the staff advocate. Look for people with expertise on the problem (e.g. other agency or "front line" human service personnel who are close to the problem), "insiders" from the target system who can look at their system objectively and who can help in understanding the power structure there, people from the community or a given profession who are influential and will be able to use their power, and allies who see the problem as you do. Additional board, staff and students can be added for their expertise or to provide advocacy training.

A good SAT member is one who is highly motivated to work on the issue. Thus, a good time to ask for volunteers is when an issue has been approved by the Advocacy Committee for an SAT. A new issue fires the imagination of advocates with ideas and hope that the situation can be changed. If insufficient people volunteer, you can think through who else should be asked with the help of a key volunteer or the chairperson you have chosen. As the SAT meets and defines the problem or sees where it needs further help, they may decide to ask someone to come for consultation on a one time, or on a regular basis. Often it will be necessary to enlarge the power base with allies from the professional community and from victims who are experiencing the problem most acutely.

Certainly if an SAT decides that it must move to a coalition of concerned professionals and community persons, the advocacy group must become much larger to represent the various aspects of the need and segments of the community. It should be organized more formally, with an executive committee and subcommittees, to work on particular areas. In coalition building it is vital to encourage the broadest participation from all segments of the community in order that all can take part in defining the basic problems.

Your enabling role begins as you invite people to join the SAT. Here you have an opportunity to infuse the prospective member with the importance of the particular advocacy issue and the need for his particular talent or expertise. You may want to discuss as well something of the agency's experience in advocating or your own conviction about advocacy as a way of helping people. Spell out the time commitment needed. (A good time interval for SAT's is to meet every other week for 1 1/2 hours or at least once a month. Duration of an SAT is more difficult to assess but you can assure the person that the SAT will decide on a timetable and readjust that if needed.) Are place and time of meeting convenient for the potential member? As you discuss these areas you can be testing for motivation to work on the issue. Be sure to leave the potential member free to decide whether this is something he really wants to do and can fit into his schedule. Gaining commitment is important so that the group will stay as stable as possible while working toward final action.

The recruit to the team may feel concern about whether to accept the risk involved in advocating. Remind him/her that this is a group effort; it is the total group who will do the study work and arrive at a consensus for action. Indicate as well that by their sanction to set up an SAT, the board of the agency sees this issue as a just cause on which to work. Point out the legal or moral rights of the group for, or with whom you will be advocating. If the potential recruit appears too hesitant, let him decline gracefully and suggest that there may be an issue in the future in which he/she will feel interested.

The recruit may feel unsure, as well, about how to advocate. You can assure him/her that we all do problem solving every day. If possible, empower the recruit by evidence of his/her problem-solving ability or instances when he/she has been helpful in the community. You can reassure the recruit that orientation to the issue will be sent to him/her in the mail (the log report and whatever additional materials are helpful), and that at the first meeting the group will receive orientation to the agency advocacy procedures and will learn together how to study and plan for action on an issue.

Should people from the offending system be invited to join the SAT? This is partly a reality, partly a strategy decision. It is probably better, in my opinion, not to invite them initially. It seems better first to be sure that the members of the SAT know clearly the nature of the problem, have adequate documentation and case evidence, and understand the target system more fully. This will enable the members of the SAT to feel greater security if they decide that the most effective initial way to seek change is to ask a member of the offending system to meet with them to discuss the problem and to share in solving it. However, in a situation where you have a reasonably cooperative relationship with people from the system where you would like change, it may be important to try problem solving together from the beginning.

Naturally, you will arrange the meeting time at the most convenient time for all SAT members to meet. This is especially important for clients or others who are experiencing the problem. Many of them will have less flexible schedules than other citizen volunteers or professionals. Sometimes it will be very difficult, or impossible, for them to come to all the meetings. If this can be recognized and accepted, but the importance of benefitting from their ideas stressed, they, and the rest of the group, can feel comfortable about this. This may happen also when so called "outside experts" are invited to the SAT on a one-time, or "come-as-often-as-you-can" basis. If the basic SAT remains consistent in its attendance, the comings and goings of those who cannot be at every meeting need not deter the total effort of the group.

People who are asked in for consultation are usually glad to be asked, but it is important for the staff advocate and the agency to remember to use their time and talent judiciously. Naturally, these consultants will need orientation to the overall goals of the group and the stage at which the particular group is. If this orientation is not done well prior to the meeting, the time of the group will be wasted in doing it.

Choosing the Chairperson

Although as staff advocate you take on the task of convening the first meeting, it is important that, if possible, a chairperson be appointed to lead the first meeting. This is less democratic, and, in terms of group process, less desirable than for the group to choose the chairperson, but my experience has been that unless a chairperson is forthcoming in that first meeting, the group tends to bond to the staff advocate as the chair, and it is both difficult for anyone else to "usurp" the role or to feel, perhaps, that he/she could do it as well. An additional problem is that members of the group might not feel in the first meeting that they know any one person well enough to assess whether that person would make a good chairperson.

Furthermore, it is important that you do not take on the role of the chairperson or secretary in order to be able to carry out your oversight and enabling roles in the SAT. The oversight role is a dual one of making sure that agency policy in the Advocacy Program is adhered to and that the advocacy process of study, selection of goals and objectives and strategies in action planning is proceeding effectively.

Not only do you not have the time to be chairperson, it is also more effective to have a board or community person as the chairperson. She/he may have more influence with community or governmental leaders. In addition, funding sources in the community will be more responsive to a citizen chairperson than to a professional; as we said earlier, professionals can be suspected of wanting to expand social services to enhance their own profession or to create jobs for colleagues. Citizens can

74

support, or withhold support, of governmental leaders, school boards, city planners and legislators.

In selecting the chairperson, look for a person with leadership qualities, who can facilitate the ideas and analytical work of the group and bring about consensus. He/she should have a stake in the issue and be capable of taking a leadership role when dialogue with the target system occurs or when confrontation, representation at public meetings or a public hearing is necessary.

PREPARING FOR THE FIRST MEETING

As staff advocate you are responsible for the seemingly humdrum details of choosing a room, date, getting together appropriate orientation materials (to the issue and to doing advocacy in the agency), setting up a file on the SAT and arranging a meeting with the chairperson to plan details of the first meeting. Although these preparations seem mundane, they make for smooth functioning of the SAT when the meeting occurs. For example, Hartford (1971:191) stresses how important the comfort and arrangement of the room is. She suggests that some spatial arrangements drive people apart, others draw people together; thus, physical arrangements may actually facilitate or impede communication, interaction and the capacity to make group decisions. Prepare wall charts and/or worksheets that show the advocacy process of study, action planning and evaluation to facilitate the advocacy work. (See discussion in Chapter Six and worksheets in Appendix 6 and 7.) A newsprint pad on which each person's ideas or the group's planning can be clearly seen will help the SAT focus on the task at hand.

Another obvious preparation is to set up a file or record for the SAT. This should include a facesheet, a list of the members of the SAT, the log and any additional information collected relating to the issue. As the work of the SAT proceeds, minutes, the initial three-month report, interim and final reports and other information will be collected in the file.

The facesheet should indicate the name of the SAT, the name of the chairperson, the log number and date of the log and the date of the initial SAT meeting. It should include also the charge to the SAT as approved by the Board on (date) and the time frame for the study phase. The following aspects can be included on the face sheet to be filled in as the study-action planning proceeds: the study-action plan (as approved by the Board on (date)), the time frame for the action phase, changes in the action plan, changes in the time frame and the date the SAT ended. A list of the participants in the SAT with their addresses and phone numbers should be affixed to the inside of the file cover for easy reference. (See Appendix 3 for a suggested facesheet form.)

Send notification of the meeting and orientation materials to SAT members well in advance. Send a map if the place or room is difficult to locate. Include the facesheet and list of participants so that they will be clear about the charge to the SAT and with whom they will be working. If necessary, send an additional notification card just prior to the meeting as a reminder.

If the group is a large one, as in a coalition, name tags are helpful, but with an SAT it is sufficient for the staff advocate or the chairperson to take the host role of making introductions and making sure that everyone is comfortable, has coffee and so forth.

Prepare a packet of orientation materials for the chairperson and each member of the SAT regarding the advocacy program structure in the agency (See Figure 1, Flow Chart for Advocacy Issues, Chapter Three) and the advocacy process of study, action planning and evaluation (See Figures 2, 3, 4, 5 and 6 in Chapter Six). Members can use these during the life of the SAT.

Prior to the first SAT meeting, plan to meet with the chairperson, not only to plan the meeting and orient him/her to advocacy but to sort out your roles and possible tasks for SAT members.

Meeting with the Chairperson

Go over the membership of the SAT; see if there are any members whom he/she feels should be added or not invited. Orient him/her to the advocacy program structure, if necessary, and the advocacy process of working on an issue to completion. Indicate that you will orient the SAT to both of these aspects of advocacy work in the first meeting and that your role in the SAT will be to keep everyone "on track" in relation to both structure and process. His/her role is to lead the meetings, to keep the group focused on the advocacy task (with your help) and to be alert to the talents and ideas of each person so that each can find, or be given a task to further the effort.

You will need to orient the chairperson sufficiently to the issue and the particular charge to the SAT so that he/she feels comfortable to begin to work on it with the SAT.

Develop an agenda for the first meeting. Self-introductions, with some time to hear why each person feels like advocating for this issue, is a good way to begin. This is helpful in practical terms of getting acquainted and in developing group cohesion regarding the advocacy effort.

The first part of the initial meeting should be allocated to training. As staff advocate, you will orient the SAT to the advocacy structure in your agency and to the steps in the advocacy process. Wall charts and a study-action packet (explained in detail in Chapter Six) showing the study-action process should be available for use by each member at the first and subsequent meetings. Such training strengthens the belief among the members that they, backed by the agency, can bring about change.

The major portion of the rest of the agenda will be taken up with a beginning look at the charge to the SAT and discussion of the problem. How this process goes will be discussed in the next two chapters.

Final items on the agenda will be discussion of a possible time frame for the study phase, frequency of meetings, adequacy of time and location and a date for the next meeting. (Note that a group contract, time frame for the study phase and measurable objectives of how many people the SAT hopes to serve are unlikely to be arrived at in the first meeting. This usually takes at least two or three meetings.)

One very important task is that of secretary. If possible, a secretary should be chosen ahead of time; if no one can be found, minute taking can be rotated among the group. This function, often considered a headache, is actually very important to the ongoing work of the SAT. Minutes keep the SAT members "on track" and inform those who could not attend a given meeting so that valuable time is not lost reorienting those who were absent. They are useful also in orienting visitors such as consultants or people from other communities who are interested in working on a similar issue in their organization. Minutes provide the ongoing record of the effort and are thus useful in evaluation, teaching, or research.

Both the chairperson and the advocate can agree to take responsibility for fostering the talents and expertise of the group either through asking for volunteers for various roles or through asking those who are less assertive. In addition to chairing and taking minutes, other tasks that SAT members can take on as the work proceeds are: <u>fact finding</u> to document need and gain general information; <u>research</u> to look for ideas for constructive change; <u>facilitating public education and public relations</u> via use of the media, being part of a speakers' bureau, preparing brochures and handouts, as well as planning or leading workshops; <u>attending various community meetings</u> related to the SAT effort; <u>researching funding possibilities</u> and thinking through the budget needs of a proposal; <u>advocating with</u>

legislators and legislative aides; and writing proposals. Other projects might require additional tasks. The point is that there are so many important tasks in advocating that each person can feel needed and important to the total effort.

It will be important to recognize the ideas, skills and feelings of the chairperson as you plan together. He/she may or may not share his anxiety about taking on the chairing of an SAT for the first time. You will need to be supportive and assure him/her of your continued backing and willingness to work with him/her for the duration of the SAT. Some chairpersons may need more shared planning time than others. The ongoing work of the SAT is usually facilitated by either face-to-face meetings or telephone conferences prior to SAT meetings.

WORKING WITH THE STUDY-ACTION TEAM

To work most effectively with the study-action team you will need to use your educational skills to orient them to the advocacy structure in your agency and to teach the advocacy process of problem solving. You will have to be aware of the overall group process: how the SAT members are (or are not) working together and how the advocacy task is proceeding. Inherent in the staff advocate's role is ongoing evaluation of whether the SAT is on track and should continue. You will also be called upon to use your enabling skills to encourage, listen to feelings, and generally empower individuals and the group to achieve its goal. In addition, you will have to keep on top of administrative tasks: filling out statistics for each meeting (see SAT Meeting Data Sheet in Appendix 4), making sure that the minutes were done and sent out, that a room was assigned, as well as keeping agency administration (the advocacy coordinator or the executive) informed of details or concerns about SAT's.

Let us look in more detail at how you will carry out these aspects of your staff advocate role as you work with the chairperson and the SAT in the first and subsequent meetings.

ORIENTATION

After introductions and a brief discussion of why the SAT has come together, the chairperson invites the staff advocate to orient the group by means of the study-action packet that is given to each member. This packet contains Figure 1: Flow Chart for Advocacy Issues (see Chapter Three); Figure 2: Steps in the First Phase of Study-Action Planning: Problem, Solution and Goal Analysis; Figure 3: Steps in the Second Phase of Study-Action Planning: Planning Strategy for Action; Figure 4: Guidelines for Evaluation of a Study-Action Team; Figure 5: Types of Intervention and Tactics; and Figure 6: Final Action Planning.

(See Chapter Six.) In addition, the packet contains worksheets for the First and Second Phase of Study-Action Planning as set forth in Appendices 6 and 7.

The staff advocate begins by explaining the advocacy structure in the agency; that is, how issues "flow" from the caseworker's log to the Advocacy Committee to the Board's sanction to set up the SAT (See Figure 1). He/she points out how the SAT will be responsible to the Board for careful study and an action plan that must be approved by the Board, prior to taking action. This will enhance a sense of stability and seriousness in the way the advocacy program is organized; it will reduce feelings of anxiety also of where the advocacy activity might lead, such as, "Will we be called upon to march on City Hall or demonstrate in the Square?" They can be assured that the latter would be reserved for extreme necessity when all other avenues of dialogue and negotiation had failed. (See Chapter Six for a discussion of strategy.)

Since the study-action packet can be somewhat overwhelming to a would-be advocate, it is important that the staff advocate put emphasis on the fact that they will use these to guide their study and action planning and that they will gradually see where each can be used at various stages of the work. The staff advocate should go over Figures 2 and 3 in some detail. Some of the advocate group may like the study-action guides, others will find the worksheets most helpful for this aspect of the process. The Guide for Evaluation introduces the idea that they will be evaluating their work as they go along and that they will have a framework within which to assess the SAT's progress.

In general, the guides aid in the orientation process by putting lay and professional persons on an equal footing as they begin problem solving; it is, thus, a shared experience rather than one in which the staff advocate takes a leader-organizer role. These guides will be discussed in detail as we think through the study-action and evaluation processes in subsequent chapters.

In addition to learning about the advocacy process, the SAT will need to educate itself regarding the issue. Especially in the early stages of study, self-education is very necessary. This could be done as needed in each meeting, or certain meetings to which outside experts or consultants have been invited could be set aside for that purpose. Much of the study, however, can be divided among members of the group, who can, in turn, educate the total group.

EMPOWERMENT

At the beginning and during the work of most SAT's that seek system change or new services, empowerment is a necessity.

Although all members presumably joined the SAT because they wanted to change what they considered to be an untenable situation, they need to feel as well that their cause is just and that they will share responsibility for study and action. Some of this belief comes from the group cohesion that develops over the issue; some comes from the belief you convey as staff advocate that through sharing ideas and willingness to risk, a committed group can solve an advocacy problem. (Refer to Chapter Two for fuller discussion of this.)

As each member feels needed and important through contributing to the study, planning and action effort with their ideas as well as fulfilling certain tasks, empowerment grows. Clarification of the SAT process and task is also empowering, as it reduces anxiety and develops skills.

Some problem areas where empowerment and education are especially needed are when the group feels overwhelmed with the task, feels stuck, or meets difficult obstacles, and has to deal with resistance. I will deal with these now under "process concerns."

PROCESS CONCERNS

Concerns regarding the process are such issues as: the role of the chairperson as compared with the role of the staff advocate, how activist the staff advocate should be, how to maintain the group and recognize individual needs, how to achieve a group contract concerning the task and how to deal with various problems that arise.

Clarification of the Roles of the Chairperson and the Staff Advocate

At times the chairperson and the staff advocate have similar roles, since they are both there to facilitate the work of the group and to keep the effort in focus. The chairperson, however, has the major role in keeping the meeting focused so that agenda items are followed and certain steps in the task are completed. The chairperson, who is usually a lay person, brings his community perspective to the task and should facilitate that among other community members in the group. He/she needs to ask such questions as: What are the constraints in this community? What will work best? As he/she listens to the ideas and concerns of the members, the chairperson should be making assessments also as to who will fill certain roles in the team work to best advantage. He/she should, of course, be able to promote discussion as well as to limit it.

With the help of the staff advocate, the chairperson should promote a group contract concerning the problem to be worked on, the goal of the effort, the tasks involved, volunteers to do the tasks, and a timetable within which completion of at least a given aspect (for example, study) is expected by the group. Such a contract will give parameters, and therefore security, within which the group can work. He/she should also push for clear objectives that are measurable, if possible, that will provide a base from which to evaluate the total effort later. (See further discussion of the task process in Chapters Six and Seven and discussion of evaluation in Chapter Eight.) In conference between meetings, the chairperson and the staff advocate should make sure that the advocacy effort is proceeding effectively and if not, why.

As I indicated at the beginning of this chapter, the staff advocate carries the professional role of representative of agency policy and advocacy skills. In addition to setting up the advocacy work, the staff advocate must operate creatively to empower the ongoing study and action planning, and to facilitate implementation of the action to a successful conclusion. She/he will enable evaluation of the work at each stage and a final evaluation on completion of the advocacy effort. As the staff advocate carries out this task in concert with the chairperson and the advocate group, she/he may have to play many roles, according to the task and the milieu in which she/he is working. The staff advocate will have to decide when it is better to delegate a task and when to assist or do it alone.

The staff advocate has the dual role of participant-observer made possible because the chairperson is carrying the ongoing functioning of the meeting. As participant-observer, the staff advocate will monitor the advocacy process. As in casework, she/he will diagnose the problem, support and empower, and suggest interventions. Some of these interventions or suggestions may be made in the group meeting and some later to the chairperson, who can implement them in the next meeting.

The staff advocate should be evaluating the ongoing work of the SAT. She/he should be looking for where changes should be made, such as enabling additions to the group (allies, people with the problem, "insiders" from the target system), recognizing the need for consultation, more information, better documentation or training in advocacy skills. He/she should be ready to deal with stalemates, offer support and empowerment. In addition the staff advocate will have to be alert to whether the executive of the agency should be involved in any (or all) of the meetings. The executive (or his designate) should be there, at least selectively, if agency policy or programs would be affected.

Another consideration for the staff advocate is how active she/he should be? The answer to this is, of course, relative to the need in any given group situation or task. My own bias is that the advocate may operate on a continuum ranging from background supporter to outright activist. Rothman (1974:75)

81

suggests that advocates have sometimes not been sufficiently assertive in their community intervention roles. He suggests that a more accurate analysis of the climate of the community may reveal that greater assertion is possible and desirable. He feels, however, that this depends on the situation, the group's goals, and the feelings of community participants. In small, informal committees the advocate should take a "more directive, task-oriented role." However, in a formal group he/she should be much less directive and especially cautious of assertiveness with target groups whose members feel distrustful, inferior or distant from the advocate. In the latter case, this caution can lessen when trust and a working relationship become established.

Rothman (1974:83) identifies three basic role orientations among professional workers: "professional orientation implies a high concern with professional values and standards, bureaucratic orientation refers to a preoccupation with policies and norms of the employing agency, and client orientation connotes a primary attention to the needs of those served by the agency." His review of the literature suggests that social workers tend to put the employing agency ahead of professional norms. He says that this tends to encourage conservatism among social workers, particularly caseworkers as compared to community organizers and group workers. His view is that client needs may suffer if administrative prerogatives are allowed to dominate and a balance needs to be struck among professional and bureaucratic orientations and client need (75). It is my own belief that an advocacy program in a casework agency, for example, attempts to redress this balance. This tends to produce, appropriately, in my view, a more activist approach on behalf of clients and of families who may never be the clients of the agency. A responsible advocacy structure can keep the bureaucratic "control" intact, but at the same time affords freedom of action within professional limits and values to both the staff advocate and the advocate group.

Maintaining Group Cohesion and Recognizing Individual Needs

An important process issue is how to maintain group cohesion and recognize individual needs as you get on with the task. I have found the concept of "M.I.T." useful. (Reference unknown.) "M" stands for maintenance of the group, "I" for individual needs of members of the group, and "T" for task. Too often, leaders of groups, lay or professional, get so involved with the task that they ignore the maintenance of the group and the individual needs of each member. This M.I.T. concept is useful for the chairperson as well as the staff advocate to keep in mind.

Maintenance of the group refers to fostering a group feeling. There are social aspects to this as well as group process aspects. Social aspects include making sure that

82

everyone has met, socializing before and after the meeting, and filling in latecomers. Fessler (1976:123) adds a number of group process tasks such as: _encouraging_ (just as in casework, the belief that there can be change is a hope that is needed by the couple or family in conflict; similarly in advocacy, the group needs the advocate's unswerving belief that the advocate task can be accomplished and that he/she will persevere whatever the ups and downs;) "_gatekeeping_" (helping the less assertive members state their ideas and restraining the over-talkative;) "_standard setting_" (using the structure under which the group operates to help the group arrive at a constructive and amicable consensus;) _summarizing group feelings; diagnosing difficulties_ and proposing possible options; _helping people to compromise_ to gain consensus; "_harmonizing_" (dealing with negative feelings;) _testing for consensus;_ and "_following_" (listening with interest as others talk.) Maintenance is the oil to facilitate the smooth running of the group machinery.

Individual needs of members are met through recognizing those ideas and feelings unique to each person (especially those who have experienced the problem), appreciating their willingness to take on tasks, affirming their potential for leadership and so forth. Since values and commitment might vary from one person to another in the group, the discussion should promote opportunities for each person to share how he feels about the issue, any doubts or concerns about the advocacy effort or his level of commitment.

Task means getting the job done! One of the important aspects of the group's work is to develop a group contract concerning the task. How this can best be achieved is really a combination of recognizing the needs and ideas of the group and using the advocacy process that we will discuss in detail in the next two chapters. This is where people and process come together in a workable plan.

PROBLEMS THAT MAY ARISE AS THE WORK PROCEEDS

The SAT Feels Overwhelmed

In the first meeting the SAT begins by discussing the advocacy problem and attempts to define it. As this discussion proceeds the group will almost inevitably find that the problem is much bigger and more complex than anyone (including the advocate) realized. The group has overturned a rock and found a host of problems underneath! The group feels overwhelmed! At this point as advocate you need to remind the group that this is a very normal phenomenon in advocacy work. An interesting way of looking at the various "normal" phases through which groups must struggle to achieve their goals is Tuckman's (1965) formulation of group process: "forming, storming, norming and performing." In order to help the group feel less overwhelmed, you and the chairperson will need to help the members partialize the problem into one with which they feel they can work. (Note the similarities to casework.)

The SAT Feels That It Is At a Stalemate

If the SAT reaches a stalemate, it is very important to have the total group discuss this. First, the group should be encouraged to ventilate its feelings of discouragement, resistance, or difference. Are the feelings realistic or do the feelings stem from a first experience with advocacy, and insufficient recognition of the ups and downs of the process? Second, why does the group feel as it does? Review where you have come from and how possible it is to do what you hope to do. Perhaps the advocacy task is impossible for this group. If not impossible, but merely difficult, how can the group get more help to get on with its task?

First, partialize the problem. Then look at the group's approach to the problem to see where they are and what they need to do. Use the study and action planning guide and the SAT evaluation guide. (See Figures 2, 3, and 4). You may need additional outside help: call on experts for more education of the SAT and/or get more ideas from libraries or other research resources (see Chapter Six). Finally, empower the group as was discussed in Chapter Two.

The SAT Has to Deal with Resistance from the System or the Community

The SAT needs to understand how and why people oppose or resist change. This is a very common problem, which will be discussed in Chapter Seven when we talk about the action phase.

Individual Versus Group Needs in the SAT

Two instances of individuals putting their needs before the needs of the group come to mind: persons who are persistently late and persons who have experienced the problem (usually personally) who need to go over and over their personal "story" of the problem whenever any aspect is discussed. Although it is understandable that some lateness will occur, it is disruptive to the "flow" of the group when latecomers must be brought up to date. Similarly, while it is very important for persons experiencing the problem to tell their story, both for its value in energizing the group to the the reality of the problem, and for its therapeutic value to the person affected, repeated telling of the story without regard to the group's goals becomes disruptive and even irritating.

When individual needs seem to be put ahead of the group process, it is incumbent upon the chairperson to discuss the problem privately, if the person is a volunteer. Similarly, the staff advocate should discuss the problem with staff or students if they are the offenders.

It is also important to clarify with members who are repeatedly absent whether they wish to continue with the SAT and to make their decision clear to the group.

ADMINISTRATIVE DETAILS

While we have focused mainly on the process, the importance of administrative details must not be overlooked. All of these are the responsibility of the staff advocate. Some are: has a room been arranged for the next meeting? Did the secretary of the SAT send in the minutes so that they could be typed and sent to each member? Is an additional notification of the meeting date needed? Has the SAT Meeting Data Sheet been filled out with statistics for the last meeting and the number of people served in the interim? Has the agenda been prepared and/or a conference held with the chairperson? Has the Advocacy Committee received appropriate reports, for example: the initial report after three months of work, the final action plan or the annual report of the SAT? Keeping on top of these administrative details will prevent misunderstanding about meeting times or places, inaccuracy in statistical findings and help in recollection of meeting details or plans.

ORGANIZING AND WORKING WITH COALITIONS

The same principles that we have discussed in relation to choosing SAT members -- high motivation to work on the issue, willingness to risk, willingness to commit to an extended time period to work on the issue -- are also true in choosing or encouraging volunteers to a coalition. It is vital in coalition building to choose people who are representative of the concern in the community, especially if the issue is controversial. It is equally important to encourage each person's participation in the work of the coalition. Thus, in planning for the first meeting, it is important that the issue be presented in a way that seeks everyone's response and in a way that does not prejudge or present a solution. The coalition needs to work together (as we have seen in the SAT) to study the issue, to develop ideas for change, to see what is a feasible goal and thus come to a plan for action. This process develops group cohesiveness and a feeling of power with which to tackle the issue.

To encourage and enlist participation at the first meeting, the focus should be on problem identification; subsequent meetings could produce tentative solutions, but it is important that the community group keep open to compromise with the decision-makers they are wanting to influence. Fessler (1976:40) cautions that if definite solutions are arrived at too quickly by people inexperienced in advocating, their solutions can seem as if they are "demands" either in the eyes of the community or to the coalition itself. This can then make compromise more difficult. What is important in initial meetings is to get a clear statement of the problem before moving to find solutions.

One way to do this with broad participation is what Fessler (1976:42) calls a "community wide", problem-identification workshop" (essentially the format described in Chapter Three in the first meeting regarding abused women.) In such a workshop people can identify the problems in small groups, and those groups can bring their findings to the total group where priorities can be set. This gives everyone the feeling that his or her view is respected and needed. If the community meeting is too large to make this feasible, a panel presentation from people representing varied points of view on the issue, followed by questions from the audience, is an alternative. Or the audience could be asked to break into "buzz groups" to share their questions and bring their findings back to the total group.

In regard to meetings on controversial issues, Fessler (1976:39) cautions that there may need to be a means to correct misinformation and supply correct information. If outside experts are brought in to meet the need for correct information, they must be people who can relate well to the local group in order that the latter can hear them. For a fuller discussion of working with controversy in large groups, and working with controversy along socioeconomic lines, see his excellent book: Facilitating Community Change.

THE ENDING PHASE

Just as you, as staff advocate, had the key role in beginning the SAT, so, too, your role in a definitive ending is important. There are three aspects to ending either a total SAT effort or a single meeting: organizational, evaluative and expressive.

The Ending Phase of a Single Meeting

Let us look first at the ending phase in a single meeting. There will be organizational aspects of what the group must do next, such as the date and time of the next meeting, frequency of meeting, the next agenda, tasks to be worked on between meetings, and adequacy of the location.

Second, there is an evaluative aspect that asks: "how well have we done today as a group?" It is here that the advocate and

the chairperson, and indeed the group members, can reinforce one
another's sense of accomplishment, purpose, and feelings of
strength to continue with the task. Everyone's effort, talent
and time should be appreciated openly. Problems that arise must
also be faced and handled. The staff advocate should encourage
the group to use the Guide for Evaluation of an SAT in Figure 4,
not only when there are problems, but at each stage of
study-action planning. Evaluation not only helps the SAT to
think about where they are and should go, but gives positive
feedback about how well they are doing that helps to energize the
group; alternatively, negative evaluation may give feedback that
forces an appropriate early termination.

Third, there is the expressive aspect, which refers to
giving group members the opportunity to share their feelings
about the meeting and the work on the issue thus far. This is
important because it fosters the affective linkages that are the
power that fuels group spirit and commitment. Positive feelings
are easily expressed and dealt with by both the advocate,
chairperson and the group members; as important as these are, it
is even more important to encourage the expression of concerns,
doubts, fears, irritations and questions of all kinds.
Professionals and volunteers, for different reasons, may feel
uncomfortable about showing "weakness" by sharing concerns, or
may feel too polite to share irritations. Thus, the advocate and
the chairperson need to be sure that these are expressed. To
facilitate a positive ending, point up the positives of this
meeting and the concerns that have been expressed. Deal with the
negatives as much as time permits. However, if more time is
needed, ask for consensus that these concerns will be placed
first on the agenda for the next meeting. Note that chatting and
socializing at the end of the meeting are important in terms of
"maintenance" of the group or meeting individual's needs; these
informal conversations can give important clues too about how
individuals feel about the work thus far or how they might be
willing to advance the effort.

The Ending Phase of a Study-Action Team

In the ending phase of an SAT or coalition, you will need to
be sure that these same aspects -- organizational, evaluative and
expressive have been covered.

Organizational aspects involve writing a final report to be
submitted to the Advocacy Committee and the Board, which will
then become part of the program report for that year. This can
be done by the chairperson, secretary, a volunteer or the staff
advocate. All members of the SAT or coalition should be informed
of the results of the advocacy effort through a copy of the final
report, a letter of appreciation, and possibly a celebration
meeting. If follow-up will be necessary, plans should be made

for how often that should be done and who, in addition to the staff advocate and chairperson, will be responsible for it.

A final evaluation of the SAT, using the Guide for Writing the Annual (or Final) Report of the Study-Action Team set forth in Figure 7 (see Chapter Seven) should be done by its members, if at all possible. This evaluation should become part of the final report. However, it is often difficult to get SAT members to come to a meeting when they feel that their work is done. In that case, an evaluation can be done by the writer of the final report and a final evaluation by the annual Program Evaluation Committee described in Chapter Eight.

The expressive aspect can be encouraged easily at a celebration meeting. List your accomplishments and those you were unable to fulfill on newsprint for all to see. Be aware that although there may be feelings of elation and relief that the task is done, the right or need met, and the dysfunctioning system changed, there may also be some feelings of letdown, and a reluctance to end the venture and to relinquish relationships among members of the group that have come to mean so much. To achieve a positive ending the staff advocate and the chairperson need to help the group "graduate" with deserved feelings of accomplishment, at the same time recognizing the very real attachments that have been built up through the advocacy experience.

When the advocacy effort ends successfully, this is easy to handle for everyone concerned. When the advocacy effort becomes impossible to continue, the staff advocate, the chairperson, or sometimes the Advocacy Committee, to whom the problem is taken, may help the SAT to end the effort. This happens occasionally during the study phase when the SAT realizes there is insufficient documentation, support or other reason to continue the effort. It is difficult for the group members, but the reality can be dealt with and the effort applauded; sometimes there will be a sense of relief.

If an SAT or a coalition has been working hard without success, particularly if they have moved to action phase, such a group will need all the recognition for a good try and support of their aims that the Advocacy Committee, the advocacy coordinator, other professionals or the group members can give. The Advocacy Committee can give recognition of the problems faced and support the SAT chairperson, advocate and group members through this painful stage. It should be stressed that the agency will look for opportunities to use their talents on other issues. The advocacy coordinator needs to be aware particularly of the needs of the staff advocate for support and recognition for what was done and the limitations faced.

Throughout this chapter we have focused on the role of the staff advocate particularly in relation to the needs and feelings of individuals and the group working on the advocacy effort. What we have indicated less is that the staff advocate sometimes is going to feel anxious, overwhelmed, stuck. He/she needs to be ready to use the support and consultation available in the agency -- with the advocacy coordinator, if there is one, or with a supervisor or the executive director. In a beginning program the staff advocate may also be the coordinator of the program. If there is insufficient consultative help within the agency, such help should be brought in or the staff advocate can educate himself/herself through books, conferences and workshops.

Let us move now to how to advocate on an issue -- the advocacy group task.

REFERENCES

FESSLER, D. (1976) Facilitating Community Change. LaJolla: University Associates.

HARTFORD, M.E. (1971) Groups in Social Work. New York: Columbia.

ROTHMAN, J. (1974) Planning and Organizing for Social Change. New York: Columbia

TUCHMAN, B. (1965) "Developmental Sequence in Small Groups." Psychological Bulletin 63.

SIX

THE ADVOCACY GROUP TASK: STUDY AND ACTION PLANNING

Responsible and effective advocacy takes an ordered, disciplined approach to social change. It requires careful study, rational planning, and repeated evaluation of the adequacy of the advocacy process and the feasibility of the goal. This is important for two reasons: first, the advocacy effort may stand or fall on the basis of one opportunity to convince representatives of a system that a change or new service is needed; second, staff and volunteer time is valuable and must not be wasted on poorly thought through efforts. In advocacy, preparation far exceeds the time spent in actual action, and for sound reasons.

THE PROCESS OF STUDY-ACTION PLANNING

We shall look first at what the SAT has to work with as it begins, namely its charge as authorized by the Board. We shall then consider in detail the steps that go into the phases of study-action planning: in the first phase, problem, solution and goal analysis; in the second phase, planning strategy for action, and finally, evaluation.

Charge to the Study-Action Team: The Task

As discussed in Chapter Four, the SAT's charge is defined initially by the motion that the Advocacy Committee makes to the Board to set up the SAT. This charge is finally rescinded, revised, or authorized by the Board. Sometimes the charge will include a beginning idea of a goal. Often, however, the goal is not clear until the SAT has studied the problem. As the SAT examines the problem in more depth, it may find that the scope of the problem as defined initially was too broad or too narrow and that it must define the charge more carefully. The goal of the SAT becomes defined after the SAT completes its analysis of the problem, the desired solution and decides on a workable goal. If the goal has been changed from the original charge, the SAT must report this to the Board and receive sanction to continue with a delimited or enlarged goal.

PHASES OF STUDY ACTION PLANNING

Let us look at the various aspects involved in study-action planning: first, problem, solution and goal analysis; second, planning strategy for action, and third, evaluation. In the first phase, problem analysis and solution analysis really amount to: what is the problem and what does your SAT want to do about it? However, problems are complex and so, too, in many cases, are solutions. Even when you pinpoint the solution you want, which then becomes your goal, you must break that down into concrete objectives. To simplify this, think of P S G/O: PROBLEM, SOLUTION (= GOAL), GOAL/OBJECTIVES (steps in achieving the goal). Figure 2 outlines the steps involved in this first phase of study. Figure 3 outlines the steps in the second phase of study: planning strategy for action. Planning strategy for action focuses on <u>interventions:</u> <u>where</u> and <u>how,</u> <u>who</u> will do it and <u>how</u> they handle it.

The Guidelines for Evaluation of a Study-Action Team in Figure 4 focus on whether the SAT is carrying out the study-action process adequately within the goals and objectives of the Advocacy Program. These guidelines are helpful to the SAT and particularly to the staff advocate and the chairperson who carry the main responsibility for evaluation.

As the staff advocate you can use these step charts as guides to orient the SAT, to educate them about advocacy principles, and as a continuing guide during the life of the SAT. The guides can be put on newsprint and placed on the wall for all to see as they work on a problem. Such "road maps" help to keep the SAT "on course". You may find the worksheets (based on these guides) in Appendix 6 and 7 helpful for each SAT member to use as you think through the problem, action plan and evaluate the ongoing work of the SAT. These charts plus Figure 5 (Types of Interventions and Tactics) and Figure 6 (Final Action Planning) can be given as a study-action packet as discussed in Chapter Five. The Worksheet for the First Phase of Study-Action Planning (see Appendix 6) could be used as a first report on study to the Advocacy Committee.

Before we look in more detail at study-action planning and evaluation, I want to remind you, if you are a caseworker reading this, of the similarities between casework and advocacy. In casework, problem-solving is done by a process of diagnosis, treatment and evaluation; in advocacy, problem-solving is done through a process of study, action planning and evaluation. Note that, as in casework, all three phases are going on at the same time.

STEPS IN THE FIRST PHASE OF STUDY-ACTION PLANNING
PROBLEM, SOLUTION, AND GOAL ANALYSIS

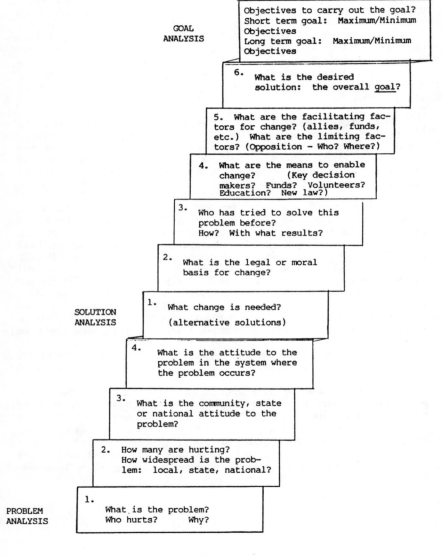

GOAL ANALYSIS

Objectives to carry out the goal?
Short term goal: Maximum/Minimum Objectives
Long term goal: Maximum/Minimum Objectives

6. What is the desired solution: the overall goal?

5. What are the facilitating factors for change? (allies, funds, etc.) What are the limiting factors? (Opposition - Who? Where?)

4. What are the means to enable change? (Key decision makers? Funds? Volunteers? Education? New law?)

3. Who has tried to solve this problem before? How? With what results?

2. What is the legal or moral basis for change?

SOLUTION ANALYSIS

1. What change is needed? (alternative solutions)

4. What is the attitude to the problem in the system where the problem occurs?

3. What is the community, state or national attitude to the problem?

2. How many are hurting? How widespread is the problem: local, state, national?

PROBLEM ANALYSIS

1. What is the problem? Who hurts? Why?

FIGURE 2

92

STEPS IN THE SECOND PHASE OF STUDY-ACTION PLANNING;
PLANNING STRATEGY FOR ACTION

AL:

TION OBJECTIVES: Short-Term Goal: maximum/minimum objectives
                   Long-Term Goal: maximum/minimum objectives

TLINE OF THE ADVOCACY CASE FOR CHANGE: (Problem definition, change needed,
goals and objectives.)

STEM ANALYSIS:
WHO are the key decision-makers who have power to make changes?
WHO on the "inside" might help to understand the system?
WHAT are some praiseworthy aspects of what they are doing?
WHERE do the system's goals and objectives match those of the advocate
     group? WHERE do they differ?
WHAT reaction can the advocate group expect:
     support? resistance? or a combination?

TERVENTIONS:
WHERE will the advocacy group intervene?
HOW will the advocacy group intervene?

    With what level of conflict: dialogue, education, negotiation or
    confrontation?

    With what tactics: letter, position paper, workshop, interview,
    media coverage, testimony, etc. (See Figure 5, Chapter Six)

HOW will the advocacy group deal with resistance?
WHO will do the intervening? SAT? Coalition? People with the problem?

ALUATION OF THE STUDY-ACTION PLAN (See Guide for Evaluation of a Study-
Action Team in Chapter Six)

NAL ACTION PLANNING (See Figure 6 in Chapter Six)
Final Preparation of the Case for Change (e.g. position paper, preparation for dialogue, workshop, etc.)

Preparation for Initial Meeting with Decisionmakers:

Meeting place, agenda, roles, content of presentation(s), preparation
via training and role playing.

TION PHASE:
ALUATION OF ACTION PHASE (See Guide to Annual (or Final) Evaluation of an
SAT in Chapter Eight)

RIFICATION OF CHANGE
RMINATION

FIGURE 3

93

GUIDE FOR EVALUATION OF A STUDY-ACTION TEAM

Conformance to Goals

Does the initial charge to the SAT (and/or the current goal) match the goals of the agency and the Advocacy Program?

Which goals of the Advocacy Program are addressed by the SAT?

Organization

Is the SAT operating within a well-defined charge (original or new

Are estimates to complete the work realistic re: people to be served, time frames, number of meetings, staff and volunteers need

Should the SAT be reorganized in any way?

Process

Analysis - Is there clear analysis of the problem, the proposed solution and the system within which the SAT seeks change?

Goals and Objectives - Are the SAT's goals and objectives clear?

Action Plan - Are there specific action objectives to carry out t goal?

If action objectives are planned, are they achievable?

Is the intervention plan appropriate to the task/situation?

Advocacy Resources - Are the needed advocacy resources available: documentation, power base, technical expertise, facilitating skill funding?

Results

Will the results be worth the effort and cost required?

FIGURE 4

94

STEPS IN THE FIRST PHASE OF STUDY-ACTION PLANNING:

PROBLEM, SOLUTION, AND GOAL ANALYSIS

Problem Analysis[1]

1. <u>What is the problem?</u> <u>Who is hurting?</u> <u>Why?</u> Usually the SAT starts with <u>a</u> problem; as they analyze it, they realize that the issue is much more complex, and that there are really interrelated problems. As discussed in the previous chapter, the problem often become overwhelming. It is therefore imperative to delimit the problem to workable proportions. The first step in this problem-solving process is for the SAT to get a clear problem statement of what is feasible for the advocacy group to work on. A <u>problem statement</u> is important because it is vital that the group <u>write down</u> (preferably on newsprint for all to see) exactly what they have agreed to work on. This is the definitive charge for the SAT's work. Moreover, it is the beginning of the contracting process discussed in the previous chapter, and it is the beginning of the problem-solving process.

2. <u>How many are hurting?</u> <u>How widespread is the problem: local, state, national?</u> <u>To what degree are people affected?</u> These are basic questions to document <u>need,</u> usually a key to the whole advocacy effort. The SAT must get facts to demonstrate need in order to convince community leaders, representatives of target systems or funding sources.

How can you and your allies document the need? Answers can be secured through service statistics (including those who may be on a waiting list), grievance and complaint data, calls for help that agencies could not meet, surveys, use of census data, interviews with clients and others who have experienced the problem, interviews with practitioners, administrators, analysis of previous studies or data, or combinations of these methods. Public hearings, community forums or meetings with any group of lay or expert witnesses, community and political leaders can provide a broader information base. First-hand information can be obtained by using observers in courts, nursing homes and so forth. (Kimmel, 1977:15)

Although there are all these methods of gaining documentation, your advocacy group must ask itself whether it has the resources to carry out a particular needs assessment method and later collate and analyze the data. The method may have to be simpler if your group is small and has no clerical assistance. On the other hand, you might find volunteers to help from among college students, another group, or people experiencing the problem.

3. __What is the community, state or national attitude to the problem?__ Who sees the problem as you do? Who sees the problem differently, as non-existent or not significant enough to be concerned about? Who will gain and who will lose if the problem remains the same?

4. __What is the attitude to the problem in the system where the problem occurs?__ First, are they aware that there is a problem? Second, if they are, would their reaction to your concern be one of wanting to cooperate in reducing or eliminating the problem? Or would their attitude more likely be hostile, either openly or passively? At this early stage in study it may be difficult to assess what their attitude would be, but if you know it now, it will have a bearing on how you think about solutions, which we shall look at next. (Note that later in the chapter we shall make an in-depth analysis of the system when we consider planning for action.)

Now that you have the data to indicate clearly the dimensions of the problem, look again at your problem statement. Is it necessary to partialize the problem and work on one part at a time? Does the problem involve many systems, and therefore you will have to choose which ones are most amenable to change? To answer these questions adequately you may have to wait until you have completed the next phase of study: solution analysis.

Solution Analysis

To get to the desired solution involves beginning with the question: what change is needed? Then the SAT must see what will enable or deter a solution by answering these questions: what is the legal or moral basis for change? Who has tried to solve this problem before? What are the means to enable change? What are the factors that will facilitate or limit change? When the SAT knows the solution they want, this becomes the overall goal for which they will work.

1. __What change is needed?__ After discussing the various alternative solutions that would help to solve the problem, the SAT must come to what it feels specifically needs to happen to eliminate the problem. The SAT may need "a better idea" as a suggestion for change. Such ideas may come spontaneously from the meeting of minds in the group, or they may have to be researched in public and university libraries, newspapers and magazines, clippings and books of the group members, the agency's advocacy resource file, or from professional organizations and research institutions relevant to the problem. It is important to keep a list of advocacy organizations that might be of help when needed. Public law centers (see Appendix 5) or the local legal aid might be extremely valuable in given situations. Federal publications can be obtained from the United States Government Printing Office or free from your congressman.

2. **What is the legal or moral basis for change?** Every organization operates under some laws, regulations or charter. Learn what these are. If necessary, obtain legal or other consultation so as to be clear how, and for what, the system can be held accountable. Change can be demanded as well on the basis of clearly identified abuse or infringement of moral or human rights.

3. **Who has tried to solve this problem before?** How? By whom were these efforts made: other agencies, community groups or people who were experiencing the problem? With what results? What were the reasons for success or for failure? Such analysis might give clues to barriers to change that are less obvious or hidden.

4. **What are the means to enable change?** Is it the awareness and cooperation of key decision-makers? Is it funding for a new service? Can the change be effected with volunteers? If so, will a coordinator be needed to recruit, train and monitor the volunteers? Will the change sought need space or a place? Is it just a change of attitude in the way service is rendered that is needed or is skill building necessary through educational workshops? Does the change require a new law or a change in the regulations?

5. **What are the facilitating factors for change?** The most important facilitating factor is the strength of the advocacy power base, those who will work in coalition with the advocate group as allies: members of other professions, people who know the problem firsthand, and aroused citizens. Other facilitating factors are the group's documented knowledge and concern about the problem, their ideas for change and how to facilitate it, their ability to organize and their persistence and patience to stay with the advocacy work. Ability to research funding sources, find volunteers or donated space may be key factors to facilitate certain advocacy efforts. Naturally, a largely positive attitude in the system where you want change makes the advocates' job much easier.

What are the limiting factors? These may be: the strength and influence of the opposition; passive resistance of the system or community; insufficient knowledge about the opposition or insufficient rapport with them; overinvolvement with the issue that causes lack of objectivity and a "we:they" stance; insufficient time or people power to get the job done; or lack of funds. In any given issue there may be many others. The point is to be clear about both the advocacy potential and limitations. If your advocacy group is knowledgeable about the limitations and can deal with them, these will not come as a surprise at the point of negotiation with the target system. If

97

the limitations far outweigh the facilitating factors, the advocacy effort may be impossible to mount and should be faced by the SAT and ended for valid reasons.

6. <u>What is the desired solution?</u> When you go through the steps of solution analysis: the changes needed, the legal or moral basis for change, what has been tried before, and looked at the means to enable change as well as what will help and hinder it, you should arrive at a <u>desired solution.</u> This, solution becomes the <u>overall goal</u> of the advocacy work. Write it out in a clear statement.

Goal Analysis

The solution or goal is likely to be made up of a number of parts: some will be achievable in the short term and some will require a longer term to accomplish. Your <u>goals</u> are the overall aim of your advocate group; your <u>objectives</u> are the specifics of carrying out these goals. Write down your objectives on newsprint as set forth in Figure 2. Set priorities in terms of which are maximum and which are minimum objectives under both your short and long term goals. If possible, state these objectives in terms that are measurable: for example, how many people will be helped and in what time period. Numbers, time frames and priorities give a standard against which to evaluate change at the end of the advocacy work.

STEPS IN THE SECOND PHASE OF STUDY:
PLANNING STRATEGY FOR ACTION

Before you begin to plan strategy and action steps, make sure that your advocacy group has a clear picture of why you are advocating. Have your group outline its "case" for change, preferably on newsprint. Your case is really made up of the group's definition of the problem, the change needed and the solution you want as embodied in your goals and objectives. This is the beginning thinking through of what you will use with the target system to promote change. (See Figure 3).

Next, analyze the system and their possible response in order to think through what interventions and tactics will work best.

System Analysis

Of primary importance in planning strategy for action is to know as much as possible about the system you will be dealing with. First, <u>who are the key decision-makers who have the power to make changes?</u> Then, to help you in your analysis, <u>who on the "inside" of the system might be willing to help you understand</u>

the key decision-makers and the <u>system</u> as a whole? Learn the chain of command. Learn the decision-makers' goals, policies, procedures, and language; learn also about the attitudes prevalent in the system that are bringing negative pressure on families. (Manser, 1973:55) Learn as much as possible about how the system operates in order to see where change is possible and who will support or oppose your advocacy group. Will the key decision-makers be likely to cooperate in a solution or to resist it?

<u>What are some praiseworthy aspects of</u> what they are doing in <u>their system?</u> As advocates who are asking for change, you will be seen inevitably as critics. To blunt this feeling and to begin your first meeting on a positive note, it will be important to look for positive aspects in the system's dealing with their clients. Then you can use these positives to "join" with the system to encourage them to work with you, just as you would help a family to join with you in family therapy. You will be building on their strengths. To achieve meaningful dialogue the advocate group must try to put themselves in the "shoes" of the system. If you can genuinely empathize with them and their problems, they are much more likely to "hear" what you are asking or suggesting. As you think about dialogue with system representatives remember use of "and" rather than "but" in framing early statements about the problem and your desired solution. (Carnegie, 1981:237) For example, if you said to a group of school superintendents, "We talked with you earlier about distributing creative ideas for working with minimally learning disabled students to regular classroom teachers <u>but</u> the handout has not reached the teachers", this could put the superintendents on the defensive. However, a more cooperative reaction might be forthcoming if you said, "We appreciated very much your willingness to listen to us at your March meeting about the need for more creative ideas for regular classroom teachers to use in working with minimally learning disabled students. We also appreciated your receptiveness to the handout our SAT had prepared for teachers, <u>and</u> we need your help in how to get this to <u>all</u> teachers. We also need your ideas about how this material could be used most effectively by them."

Ask yourselves: <u>where do the system's goals and objectives match those of the advocate group</u>, and <u>where do they differ?</u> The meeting ground between you will be where your objectives and goals meet those of the system. Thinking through this positive side will help you work <u>with</u> them on solutions to the problem. However, you need to be aware equally of where their goals <u>differ</u> from those of your advocate group. If you are clear about the negatives you might receive, you will not be surprised or as likely to be defensive when you negotiate.

Finally, <u>what reaction can the advocate group expect from the system?</u> Will they be supportive, resistant or more likely supportive on some of your objectives and resistant on others? How to deal with various negative reactions will be discussed in Chapter Seven. Think through how you will react and role play ways to deal with the system's reactions. Have some of your group act as observers to critique your performance.

Interventions

Where will the advocacy group intervene in the system? At what level: head of the organization or head of a department concerned with your issue? Who are the key decisionmakers? Who is most likely to listen to your "case" for change? Would it be more feasible to begin with a part of the system rather than to try to influence the whole system?

How will the advocacy group intervene? With what level of conflict will it be best to intervene: dialogue, education, negotiation or confrontation? Depending on the probable response of the target system, the advocate group will want to consider one or more of the following types of interventions and specific tactics to implement them. See Figure 5 which draws in part from Brager and Specht (1973:272). The interventions listed begin with the least pressure and end with assertive tactics that, from the stance of a community agency, might, or might not, be applicable in doing advocacy.

Think about the probable response of the representatives of the target system. If they would be in basic agreement, the advocate group would consider dialogue: sitting down to discuss the problem and arriving at an agreed-upon plan for change. If the likely response would be fear or hesitancy, dialogue would be the intervention of choice, with shared problem solving and education as the preferred tactics. If it appears that the system would have a lack of awareness of the problem and possible solutions, education might be the intervention to use. Education can take place in many ways: through letters, position papers, workshops, articles, booklets or other handouts, media coverage, testimony and so forth.

If, however, the target system's representatives would be more likely to disagree with the need or resist doing anything about it, proposals or demands could apply sufficient pressure to produce negotiation between your position and theirs. If the system's representatives refuse to talk to the advocate group, confrontation might be necessary through use of the media, legal action or public demonstrations to bring them to the point of sitting down to dialogue or negotiate.

We will discuss possible interventions and tactics in more detail in Chapter Seven where we shall look at the action phase.

100

TYPES OF INTERVENTIONS AND TACTICS

Interventions	Tactics
	Problem Solving
	Joint Action
DIALOGUE	Education (within target group)
	Persuasion
	Lobbying
	Education (within target group)
	Education via: media, news-letters, public hearings
EDUCATION	Lobbying
	Press Conferences
	Testifying before a Legislative Committee
	Proposals
	Demands
NEGOTIATION	Bargaining
	Education (within target group)
	Negotiation
	Newspaper reports of situation
	Other media coverage — Documentary
	Press Conference
	Demands
CONFRONTATION	Lobbying
	Legal Action
	Demonstrations
	Threats of Disruption
	Boycotts

FIGURE 5

101

Who will do the intervening? Who would be the most effective intervention group? Would one or two people be best, or does it need a team who represent the SAT or coalition? Can people who have experienced the problem be involved? Would it be best to have the full SAT or coalition present? All of these considerations depend on whether you need to have a visible power base or whether key advocates will represent this power and be more acceptable and effective. Only a few people can do the talking in any case, and these should be your most effective spokespersons.

The lead presenter should be the most influential person in the eyes of the system people. This person, or the chairperson of the advocate group, could take the role of "host" for the advocate group, introducing them to the system people and giving the credentials and/or titles of each person. Be sure that the presentation team has one or two advocates with good diplomatic skills who can be effective in dealing with tense areas or hostility. If confrontation will be needed, who will be most skilled at doing this? If education will be needed, who can "teach" with a few cogent points? While the presenters are talking, there should be one member of the team who is taking notes and one or more who are observing the process and acting as resource persons. They should be ready to make suggestions about next steps for the target system or points missed by presenters when discussion or questions intervened.

Now that the action plan has been thought through, take time to look back and evaluate the job you have done.

Evaluation of the Study-Action Planning

This is the point at which the advocacy group looks back over all its work to see if it is fully prepared to take the action steps and if, in fact, the advocacy goal is achievable and worth the effort. See Figure 4: Guidelines for Evaluation of a Study-Action Team for the major areas that need to be reviewed.

If the evaluation is positive, it is time to make specific preparations for the action phase.

Preparation for the Action Phase

Simple questions to ask here are: what will you do first, second and so forth? When will you act? Who will take which roles and tasks? How will you prepare for the advocacy intervention? To answer the first two "what and when" questions, look at your objectives and schedule the advocacy actions on a timetable. Include who will take which role or task. Put this action plan on newsprint using a framework similar to the chart in Figure 6, Final Action Planning, or use a copy of that chart as a worksheet for each member of the SAT. Of course at this point only the projected numbers can be inserted. After the action phase, the actual time frame and number of people served can be added when this same form is used as a part of the final SAT report. (See Chapter Eight).

When the final action plan has been completed, the staff advocate (or a member of the SAT) takes it to the Advocacy Committee for their review and approval. The chairperson of the Advocacy Committee will then take it to the Board for their sanction. Note that the operating parameters of the SAT are now the goal and objectives as set forth in the Final Action Planning form (Figure 6) rather than the original charge to the SAT.

When these steps are completed, the SAT is ready to prepare for the initial action steps. Examples of action steps are: holding workshops, developing a newspaper article or TV program with the help of local media people, meeting with key decision-makers in a system (or community) to ask for change and/or funding of a new program, or meeting with legislators regarding passage of a new law.

Obviously, this is the time for more definitive development of your advocacy position -- the "case" for change. Depending on your intervention, this might be a position paper, a fact sheet for legislators or it might involve specific preparation of parts of what you want to do by several members of the advocacy group. Workshops, for instance, will need several presenters, discussion leaders, and so forth. Since meeting with decision-makers is needed very frequently, we shall discuss that in some detail.

Preparation for Initial Meetings with Key Decision-Makers

With the overall action plan outlined and your case for change well developed, you are now ready to prepare for your first meeting with those who are in a position to bring about change in the target system. First, prepare an agenda. This agenda should include: a) problem, b) documentation, c) possible solution(s), d) action steps. Review who will take the role of host, lead presenter, observer, resource person, notetaker and so forth. Decide who should contact the system representatives: the chairperson or possibly someone on the SAT who has a link with that system or a particular representative. Decide also whether it is strategically better to meet in your building or theirs. If someone inside the system supports you, decide whether it is appropriate to ask that that person be invited to the meeting.

Since the action phase begins with the initial telephone contact with the system representative, we will begin our discussion of the action phase at that point in the next chapter.

FINAL ACTION PLANNING

STUDY-ACTION TEAM: _____

GOAL: _____

PLANNING DATE: _____

DATE OF BOARD APPROVAL: _____

ACTION OBJECTIVES:

Short Term: Maximum _____

Minimum _____

Long Term: Maximum _____

Minimum _____

ACTION PLAN

| Action Steps | Time Frame | | Person(s) Responsible | Role/Task | People Served | Advocacy Resources | | | | | Rating by PS |
	Proj.	Act.			Proj. Act.	D	PB	TE	FS	$	0-5
1.											
2.											
3.											
4.											
5.											

Proj. – Projected
Act. – Actual

N/M – Non-Measurable
N/Ach – Not Achievable

Advocacy Resources: D – Documentation, PB – Power Base, TE – Technical Expertise, FS – Facilitating Skills, $ – Funding, PS – People Served

Rating: 0-1 Unacceptable; 2 Fair; 3 Good; 4 Excellent; 5 Outstanding

FIGURE 6

104

EXERCISE

Use the following log (or one of your own) to think through study-action planning and evaluation. Use the worksheets in Appendices 7 and 8 and charts of Figures 2, 3, 4, 5 and 6 to guide your work. This exercise can be used equally well with board and staff members or with students. Groups should be no larger than eight. Since the process could involve many hours in actuality, the exercise will have to be time limited, perhaps one half of the time for the phase of study-action planning, and one half for the second phase: ideally, one hour at the least, and two hours at the most.

If the time is limited, you might have to encourage the group to process only the first phase. The point is to give them an experience of advocacy. In one of my first experiences of a workshop on advocacy we were required to choose an issue, reach a solution and a primary intervention in 20 minutes. In such a case your questions to the group would be: What is the problem? What is the best solution to it? How can you achieve it?

ADVOCACY LOG

FAMILY SERVICE AGENCY   LOG NO. 85 Ed.

DATE: LOGGED BY: D. Smith
SYSTEM DYSFUNCTION: Education   UNMET NEED: Appropriate
                                            educational program

CASE SITUATION:

Problem: Many adolescents are referred for counseling around their attitudes to be in school. Many want to drop out -- "hate school." Some are truant or absent. Parents find difficulty in "making" them go to school.
Action Taken (or Attempted) Within System: Counseling to allow ventilation of negative feelings, support of parents and consultation with school officials and teachers is often only partially successful, sometimes not at all. Many drop out as soon as possible.

ADVOCACY PROBLEM: Who hurts? Why?

Many of these adolescents feel that school is irrelevant to their future life of work and making money. Many have poor verbal skills, but do have better, or good, performance skills. Many are interested in training for a skill at

105

students with higher academic records.

Since Vo-Tech "slots" are at a premium, vocational school administrators fear that taking a student who has been missing school, has poor motivation and a poor academic record is too big a risk.

REQUEST TO THE ADVOCACY COMMITTEE

To seek permission from the Board to set up an SAT to study the possibilities for improved educational programming that would meet the needs of students with high performance skills but low verbal skills to develop marketable work skills and to advocate for such educational opportunities.

NOTES

[1]This schema for problem solving owes much to Cox, Fred M., et al. (1970) Strategies of Community Organization. Ithaca, Ill.: Peacock.

REFERENCES

BRAGER, G. and H. SPECHT (1973) Community Organizing. New York: Columbia.

CARNEGIE, D. (1936. Reprint Carnegie D.D. and D. 1981) How to Win Friends and Influence People. New York: Simon and Schuster.

KIMMEL, W. (1977) Needs Assessment: A Critical Perspective. Washington: Department of Health, Education and Welfare.

MANSER, E. (ed.) (1973) Family Advocacy: A Manual for Action. New York: Family Service Association of America.

Seven

THE ADVOCACY GROUP TASK: ACTION

After all your study and strategic planning, it is time for action. In this chapter we shall look at how the action phase begins with the first contact with a system decision-maker. We shall then discuss how the initial meeting should be conducted using a dialogue intervention. Since systems will respond in a number of different ways, we shall look at how to match interventions and tactics to particular system responses. The chapter goes on to deal with verification that the changes desired have taken place and termination of the SAT. Finally, we shall consider how the SAT can evaluate its work and end with a final report.

THE CONTACT

The chairperson, or whoever has been designated, begins the action phase by contacting the key decision-maker in the system by telephone. This call can be relatively brief since he/she does not want to get into a premature discussion of the problem. The caller should introduce himself/herself and whom he represents, outline the concern briefly and ask for a time to talk about it. Depending on the action plan, the caller may want to discuss which people from the system should be there. She/he will also need to determine the length of the meeting time and where to meet: usually one and one-half hours is adequate. The caller should indicate that he/she will follow up with a letter to introduce the advocate group and to outline the problem a little further.

The follow-up letter should begin with how much the advocate group appreciates the opportunity to talk with the other system people. Elaborate on who the advocates are and why they are concerned about the problem. Confirm the meeting time, place and names of the participants. Enclose materials that are pertinent to the problem that would be useful to prepare for the meeting.

Prior to the meeting, review the content of your position and the materials that you will use to present it: fact sheets, charts, and possible handouts. Rehearse how the meeting will go. Discuss the best strategies. Role play while several people critique the performance.

THE INITIAL MEETING WITH REPRESENTATIVES OF THE SYSTEM

As we have indicated, your advocacy group could be at the initial meeting in full force or send a core group. In either case, a small group with predetermined roles will present. If you are the lead presenter, you should begin by introducing the advocate group to the system representatives and giving the advocates' credentials as well as the titles of the system people. Be friendly; make some small talk and try to ease into the "business" of the meeting with appreciation for the time and interest shown by the system people in being willing to sit down and talk with your group.

A positive way to begin is to praise some aspect of the system's functioning that is particularly helpful to people you know. This gives the system a reputation to live up to and begins the "joining" process. Then go on to introduce why you are there with something like: "We've appreciated . . . (spell out some areas of agreement or positive actions) . . . and we're sure you will want to work with us to find a solution to . . . (spell out the problem briefly)." At appropriate points various members of your presentation team can pick up the discussion of the problem with the aspects for which they have taken responsibility. Show where their goals and yours are similar and how the change that you are suggesting will be a "win:win" situation. (This is a situation where both sides win and there is no loser.) Find areas of agreement and try to get the system people to say "yes, yes" early in the discussion.

If it is a large group to whom you are presenting your case, you may want to do that first, then discuss. However, if the group is small and informal, discussion or questions will intervene, so that it is important to be sure that you have covered all the parts of your presentation. Advocates who take an observer role can make sure of this.

When should ideas for a solution be introduced? If the idea for solution can come from the system people they are much more likely to implement it. If one of your presenters must suggest the solution he might say something like: "This possible solution has occurred to us, but what is important is what will work for you and your clients. What do you think about this idea? (Discussion) What do you think would be the best solution?" What you are trying to do here is to let them mull over the idea, refine it, modify it, and finally take ownership so that they will be ready to implement it.

If there is resistance to your ideas, try honestly to see the system's point of view. Respect their viewpoint even if you cannot agree with it. Point to the fact that the differences between you are only of <u>method</u> not purpose. Recall areas of agreement and appeal to the high aims of their organization or their aims as professionals. Always protect their dignity and allow them to save face, if necessary.

Sum up the Results of the Meeting

Go over what has been said, pointing to specific areas of agreement. Show genuine appreciation wherever possible and underline comments of specific individuals among the system group that support the advocates' position or new ideas that have surfaced to deal with the problem. If the system people are very supportive, suggest a joint working committee to continue to work on solutions and set a meeting date to do this.

If the system people are somewhat supportive but still questioning, outline what has been accomplished and what remains unresolved. Try to work out a plan of what the system feels ready to do and perhaps how your advocate group could help. Recognize openly the uncertainties that the system people may have about both the problem and the solution, perhaps indicating some of your own concerns when you were beginning to study the problem. It is important to remember that what you are talking about may be a completely new idea to them and they will need time to think through the implications for their organization. It is often wise to postpone action to give both sides time to think through the problem and the solution. Set another meeting date or a date by which your advocate group expects to hear from the system.

As a result of the first meeting advocates often see a side of the problem and obstacles to solution that never occurred to them in the "ivory tower" of their study phase. You may have to research more ideas or think through how you can deal with the obstacles presented. You can often be more genuinely sympathetic to the system's problems than you were heretofore.

After the meeting, send a letter to the system thanking them for the time spent with them and outlining what both groups arrived at and what future plans include. Even if the system was unyielding, a letter will make it a matter of record and underline your determination as advocates.

There are several purposes for this initial meeting. Most desirable would be to have the system agree readily to make the change needed. Also desirable is to have the system agree to have representatives work with your advocacy group to bring about the change. However, if the system people are not cooperative, are resistive or fearful, the initial meeting will give your advocates useful diagnostic information about where the system people are in their thinking. Furthermore, if the system people are hostile, the initial meeting gives your advocate group the opportunity to indicate your firm resolve to pursue your objectives. As advocates you will be clear also that you have to be more confrontive in your tactics in this latter case.

INTERVENTIONS TO CONSIDER IN VIEW OF THE SYSTEM'S RESPONSE

Now, let us look at the system's response in more detail to ascertain the type of intervention and tactics that can be used as a result of knowledge gained from the initial meeting.

INTERVENTIONS AND TACTICS

Refer to the types of interventions and tactics set forth in Figure 5 (See Chapter Six). You will recall that Figure 5 is part of the study-action packet given to your advocacy group at the beginning of the SAT. Use it now to stimulate their thinking about options available to them: note that the list of tactics begins from the least pressure to the most confrontive tactics.

Some interventions, such as dialogue and education, that involve the least pressure will be a part of almost every advocacy effort. Dialogue is talking face to face about a problem as described above in the initial meeting. Education is an intervention to change attitudes and give new ideas. It is often the first step toward changing policies and practices. The amount of education needed will depend on both the degree of awareness and depth of understanding of the problem, and the degree to which the target system is aware of, and willing to consider other ways of dealing with the problem.

Many of these tactics can be used at various levels of intervention. It is the degree of pressure that is applied as much as the tactic itself that determines in which type of intervention it might be used. For example, letter writing can be either confrontive or primarily educative, as can lobbying. "Going public" through the press, public hearings or use of the media can educate or escalate the level of confrontation, depending on how it is used.

Let us look at possible ways your advocacy group could deal with various responses from systems.

110

System Responses:

Cooperative: If a positive response regarding the need is forthcoming, encourage the system's representatives to join in problem solving with your advocate group. Remember that the people in the system who are new to thinking about the problem will have to repeat the problem solving analysis that you have already done in order to be as convinced as you are. As in casework, do not do it for them, rather work together to come to a solution that feels right to everyone. It may, in fact, be a better solution than the SAT's original solution. This group will have the advantage of people who know the system and its problems first hand.

The system people, though cooperative, may want to work on the problem on their own. However, if educational efforts such as consciousness raising or skill building are needed by their staff, your group could offer to provide this or work with them to seek specialists. However, if the system appears to be overworked and says that they have little time to deal with your suggestions, be ready to suggest alternatives or your willingness to help one of their staff in researching these.

Hesitant or Fearful: If the system's representatives are hesitant, help them to think of making one small change. Then reinforce indications of beginning to think differently by positive support. Help them think of long-run positive outcomes such as positive public relations, greater visibility and positive use of private or government funding. If one of your objectives is accepted, applaud this and move to the next objective where there might be a chance of agreement.

If they are fearful, help them to discuss why. Diagnose why they feel as they do, then offer to work with them to overcome the difficulties. Work together to think through the most effective strategies and tactics.

Finally, if they continue to be hesitant, discuss the worst case scenario if nothing is done: what this would mean to their clients or constituents and how their system would be viewed.

Resistant: Some measure of resistance is often encountered in advocacy. Dealing with resistance is similar to dealing with hesitation. Diagnose where the resistance is coming from through discussion of how they feel about the problem and the solutions proposed. Biklen (1974:70-80) suggests that people oppose or resist for the following reasons. They <u>feel unable to risk:</u> perhaps because of their basic personality, perhaps for reality reasons such as fear of job loss or what people that they know would think. They <u>feel unable to change:</u> "We have always done it this way." (Advocates need to remember that change is difficult and often threatening since it always means going against the

familiar and against procedures that have been established.
Think how you would feel if some group came to suggest a series
of changes in your program or agency. Show them how they can
take one positive step and build on that to encourage more steps
in change.) They identify with a profession and see that as the
best way to do things. They identify strongly with an
institution and resent criticism of it. They feel overwhelmed by
the task. "So much needs to be done: where do we start?"
(Again, show them how they could start with one small step
ahead.)

In addition to knowing why, advocates need to be alert to how
people resist change. Biklen (1974:82–83) says systems use ploys
such as: the cover-up -- the official description of programs and
services may be very different from what is really happening.
(Find out what the real situation is.) Double talk -- "I agree
with your philosophy but . . . " where your ideas are seen as
impractical. (Challenge them to act on their beliefs and show
leadership.) Passing the buck -- "I agree with you but I am not
in a position to make the decision." (Find out who is legally or
administratively responsible for decisions. Then, if they
continue to pass the buck you could make a public issue of it.)
Another passing the buck ploy is to say "we don't have the
money." (Actually it depends on how the dollars are allocated.)

Sometimes the system people may use the following
diversionary tactics. They say that the expert knows best.
(This is used to make lay people feel less qualified to make
judgments.) They blame the victim. For example, welfare clients
are said to be cheaters who do not want to work. This leads to
doubt that anything can be done. (It is important, therefore, to
look at the total situation to see the real problem.) They blame
the advocate. Advocates are made to feel "pushy" even when they
are within their rights. The system representative says: "Your
cause is only one of many that we have to consider." Or, "You
are too involved.:" (This is where the objective study by a
group is a plus.) They keep the rules of the game undefined.
"If they can use vague terms and laws to justify their actions
organizers and advocates will have a difficult time holding them
accountable." (Biklen 1974:80) (Clarify the law or policy and
hold administrators accountable).

Sometimes system or community people wittingly or unwittingly
resist when they attack the wrong problem. Charity minded "do-
gooders" may block change by raising money for symptoms rather
than looking at the whole problem and the underlying causes.
(For example, churches stock food banks when the real need is
adequate welfare grants. This approach fills in the gaps
(sometimes a necessary one in the short run) instead of
establishing a right.)

The important point here is not to take resistance as an

affront to your position as advocates. Deal with resistance as you would in therapy: understand where it is coming from (fear or inertia), then encourage and support signs of change and evidence of dealing with it differently.

Passively resistant: System representatives can react with passive resistance as well. This may be expressed by not following through on responsibility for next steps in carrying out a goal, by failing to attend meetings or other evidence of lack of cooperation. Such behavior should be confronted and the reasons for it discussed. Diagnose whether this is resistance out of fear or covert hostility and deal with it as discussed under "resistance" or "hostility". Whichever turns out to be the case, the fact that the system people handled their anger passively suggests that they find it very difficult to tell you what they really feel, and you are going to have to help them feel able to share their real feelings.

Hostile: If the system's response is hostile, you will need to use your casework and advocate skills to reduce hostility. Begin by clarifying in an accepting tone what you hear them saying. Stay as calm as possible remembering that it is crucial to allow the system representatives plenty of time to express their negative feelings before they will be able to "hear" what you want them to deal with positively. As they are doing this, each member of the advocate group can be thinking through constructive ways to deal with their concerns or negativism. An important skill here is "reframing": move the discussion along by reframing some of the negative comments into more positive ones. For example, "is it possible that your concern about . . . might actually be less than you are thinking right now, and that . . . positive results might occur if . . . were done?"

Hostile reactions, of course, come from feeling threatened, criticized or even cornered. Help the system representatives to discuss these feelings, accepting them as understandable and natural. Indicate that you see many positives in what they are doing and appreciate those, but bring the focus to the client problem that concerns you both. To involve them in problem solving, ask what ways they see that might more effectively serve the clients in the light of the concern that you present? Encourage them to "brainstorm" solutions with you, then go over those to come to a workable solution.

If these approaches do not succeed in a move toward dialogue, move into a negotiating or confrontational framework. To promote negotiation, submit a proposal that the system people can read and consider, spelling out the best and worst case. Another way to assert the group's rights and to educate regarding a need is to formulate a list of demands. These can take the form of a "bill of rights" or a list of grievances or needs. Finally, a willingness to negotiate may come only as a result of a successful confrontation, which we shall discuss shortly.

Prior to negotiation, assess your position and theirs: what kinds of rewards or punishments can your group give? A punishment that an individual or a system might want to avoid would be public embarrassment through the newspaper; thus, threat of publicity might be sufficient to move them to negotiation. A reward a system might want to have would be enhanced prestige and positive publicity for beginning an innovative program.

Negotiation requires particularly careful preparation: goals must be clear in order to maintain cohesiveness of your advocate group, and in order not to be deflected by possible divide and conquer tactics of the system representative. Goals must be clear as well in order that your group is in agreement on the minimum for which you will settle, since in all probability not all of your demands will be met. Rehearsal becomes of paramount importance, too. Who will take which roles and undertake particular arguments? Maintain cohesiveness of your advocate group by frequent meetings in between negotiation sessions, to air concerns and feelings and to plan continuing tactics.

Above all, be clear about the advocate stance: to expect change and facilitate it. Advocates must be firm about the legitimacy of the cause and the need for change at the same time as they show understanding of the difficulties experienced by the person(s) being asked to change the system. However, this "understanding" should not go so far as to preclude pressure on the system (Brager and Specht, 1973:307). Understanding needs to be used for building a willingness to work together, or if this is not possible, to know where more, or different, pressure is needed. Biklen (1974:37) says that, as allies of the victims, advocates cannot maintain a close relationship with the victimizer. However, Sunley (1970:351) cautions that even when the offending system becomes the adversary, it should not be seen as the enemy. Advocates must keep a balance between expectation of change and awareness of the system's position.

If negotiations drag on with no definite response, Biklen (1974:109) suggests that advocates tell officials they want a definite decision within a specified time. If they are unwilling to agree to an appropriate timetable, alternative strategies that involve a more confrontive stance should be developed.

Confrontation applies the most pressure to a system. The least confrontational tactic might be use of the media: ask a newspaper reporter to do a story on the problem or discuss the situation on radio or TV as objectively as possible. The more the finger is pointed at where change should occur and who should make it, the more confrontational the tactic becomes. Press conferences, demands, legal action, demonstrations, threats of disruption or boycotts are all tactics in the confrontation repertoire. However, two cautions are important here. First, too much pressure or ill advised pressure may win the battle, but lose the war! In moderate sized communities where you and your agency are well known, too much pressure may be viewed as too radical, and give the agency and the advocate group a bad name. It is important to remember that in the future the agency and other community professionals who support you will want to work on other advocacy issues. Also, today's adversaries may be tomorrow's allies on a different issue. A second caution is that advocates in an agency that has other direct service programs such as family counseling, adoption or family life education must be mindful of the effect of their advocacy tactics on the total agency program. If as advocates you gain one needed service while losing another, what has been achieved? Remember, what happens to clients is what is most important.

In spite of the limitations on an agency that must go on living in the community, there are ways an agency can be part of a pressure group. Coalitions provide an excellent answer to this dilemma since the resulting pressure will be shared by a larger number of organizations. The initiating advocate agency can take a lower profile in a coalition, but continue to use its advocacy skills to strengthen the effectiveness of the coalition. In addition, agencies can support the legal confrontation of other organizations with position papers and documentation of the problem.

The most extreme actions under the broad classification of confrontation are legal action, demonstrations, threats of disruption and boycotts. These are more extreme than I am prepared to discuss here. Readers who are interested in such tactics should consult Biklen or Brager and Specht.

When your advocate group is convinced that the action phase is complete, it will need to allow time for the system to make changes or the new service to develop its program. Although the time interval may vary, six months is often an appropriate interval to wait to verify that the changes desired are, in fact, being implemented. Let us look now at ways to do this.

VERIFICATION OF CHANGE

Methods by which to verify change will vary according to whether the change sought is related to a dysfunctioning system, a new service, a new law, or attitude change and skill enhancement.

Dysfunctional System

In the case of a dysfunctional system, you will need to

arrange a follow-up meeting of the original SAT or coalition to to assess whether they see a change in the way the system functions. If not, or if the change is incomplete, a follow-up meeting with the target system will be necessary. The follow-up meeting might be with the SAT or coalition where that group usually meets, or it might be more effective to ask to meet at the target system's headquarters. In certain cases, an on-site visit will be essential to verify change. For example, in working to bring about shorter lines and seating for unemployment insurance claimants, verification of seating arrangements, and the length of the lines would be necessary.

At the outset of such a follow-up meeting, recognize with positive comments any changes that have been made. As is true in casework, so in advocacy it is also true that next steps in change might not happen at once. Use skills for dealing with resistance to change discussed earlier. Be open to ways your advocate group could support the decision-maker in his desire to change. If, for example, she/he is experiencing difficulty in convincing her/his associates of the validity of the change requested, she/he might welcome a "push" from your group. You might assert, for example, that you would have to go to the newspaper if nothing is done.

If no appreciable change has taken place, call your advocate group together. Determine whether they wish to continue to work on the problem. If so, analyze why change has not come about, and rethink your action plan. The following questions will help to do this:

What unexpected problems or barriers have arisen?

Is more research for alternative solutions needed?

Are different objectives needed?

Are different interventions, tactics or strategies required?

Are there sufficient resources of people (power base), dollars and technical skill to continue to facilitate the advocacy effort?

Does the advocacy group feel sufficiently empowered?

Are the desired results attainable?

Are the results worth the effort required?

New Service

Let us assume that your advocacy group was successful in bringing about a new service. To assess the adequacy and impact of a new service, client statistics and client surveys can be used to answer the following questions:

1. How many people were served? directly? indirectly?

2. How effective is the service offered: from the client's point of view? from the system's point of view?

3. Is there evidence of impact on the community? How?

4. Is information available from which to determine whether the cost benefit ratio is justified?

5. Is the service permanent?

Other means of answering these questions might be through an on-site visit, attendance at a board meeting, or a meeting between the advocate group and the director of the new service.

If there is serious doubt that a service is adequate, or that a system has changed, call a meeting of people who are experiencing the problem to assess where the gaps in service are. Those most affected might be able also to give practical ideas about what would work better for them.

Attitude Change or Skill Enhancement

Advocacy efforts that intend to produce changes in attitude or increase skills will usually use workshops, in-service training sessions, forums and so forth. Usually, evaluations are completed by the participants at the end of the workshop. You will find results of these can be useful, at least in determining the initial reaction of the participants. It will not guarantee change. You will need to observe how this consciousness-raising plays out in a given profession or system to determine the effect. Another indication of the effect of advocacy might be requests for similar workshops or forums by related groups, such as teachers who heard about a workshop given for guidance counselors and asked for a workshop for their school district.

TERMINATION

Your advocacy effort ends when you have verified that the change you want has been made. This could be when functioning of a system has improved, when a new service has begun, when educational efforts can be taken over by another organization, or when a law has been passed.

In advocacy efforts with dysfunctioning systems, it is often conducive to good relations to indicate your desire as advocates

117

to be held equally accountable for your service to people. You could ask for constructive criticism since a system outside your own may more readily see changes that would improve your program. This can cement the "we win: you win" stance. When one is advocating it is interesting how many times one sees problems in one's own agency or a fellow advocate experiences the same insight about her/his agency. Thus, there can be self-learning and change on the part of advocates as well as the identified "problem system."

When the advocates' work has been successful, celebration is in order. As discussed earlier, there may be some feeling of letdown after all the push to achieve a goal finally succeeds. To offset this, and to use their knowledge, advocates should be used in the new service as volunteers, perhaps on an advisory board or on a funding search committee for future needs. Depending on their expertise, advocates can also be used as training resources for new staff. If the advocates do remain in close touch with the new program, it is easier to determine whether the service is carrying out the appropriate function envisioned by the founders. If advocates do not have a place in the new service, they need to be reminded that they will be called on again in future efforts. Very often awareness of their skills and devotion means that they will be asked to serve on another board or community committee.

In those advocacy efforts that focus primarily on change of attitude or learning new skills, continuing education will need to be transferred to the appropriate resource to do this. For example, educational and consciousness-raising efforts might begin in your advocacy program, but, if continuing education is needed, be referred to your family life education program or some other organization in the community that is responsible for education in that system.

When the change desired is implemented, it is extremely important to thank all those who have brought this about: decision-makers, legislators, funding sources, volunteers, and your advocate group. Where community support has been crucial, it is important to recognize this by a letter to the editor or in a newspaper article about the new service.

Unfortunately, some advocacy efforts must terminate without success or with only partial success. Again, appropriate letters of thanks should be sent.

As we indicated in Chapter Five, ending an SAT involves organizational as well as expressive and evaluative aspects. Refer to that chapter for a more complete discussion of the staff advocate's role in this stage. Here let me remind you of some essential organizational steps that will help with the overall evaluative task. If possible, call a final meeting of the SAT to

GUIDE FOR WRITING THE ANNUAL (OR FINAL) REPORT OF THE STUDY-ACTION TEAM

me of Study-Action Team: Report Year:

riod Covered in Report:

mbers of SAT: (name - board, staff, community organization or special expertise)

nsultants: (name, expertise) ____No. Staff: ____Total No. Volunteers: ____board;
            ____community. No. of Meetings: ____ Total Meeting Hours: ____
            (staff ____, volunteers ____)

iginal Charge to SAT: (See SAT Face Sheet)

rrent Goal of SAT (if changed)

OCESS: Outline briefly the SAT's analysis of the:

        -Problem (including documentation and the attitude of the system to the
             problem)
        -Solution desired (including facilitating and limiting factors)
        -Goal and Objectives to carry out the goal (Short Term: maximum/minimum--
             Long Term: maximum/minimum)
        -System

tach the Final Action Plan on whichthe SAT has set forth goals, objectives, and
tion steps. On the Final Action Planning form fill in "Actual" columns with num-
rs, N/Ach for Not Achievable, or PL for Planned.

e the following advocacy resources available to further the action steps:
cumentation, power base, technical expertise, facilitating skills, funding?

SULTS

re the action objectives to carry out   Were non-measurable results significant?
e goal achieved?
                                                Were secondary gains valuable for the
s the SAT's goal achieved?   agency? for the community?

re the estimates of people to be   Were the results worth the effort and
rved, time frames, staff and   cost required?
lunteers needed for completion
 the work appropriate in terms   Was the process well done even if results
 actual results?   were poor or nil?

re measurable results significant?   How is the advocacy effort perceived
                                                by the people served?

TE: Include the SAT's subjective evaluation of its efforts and narrative comments
     that would enhance understanding of the SAT's work or inability to complete
     the goal. If this is an annual report, use those sections of the Guide that
     are applicable to the SAT's work currently.

FIGURE 7

119

sum up and evaluate results. Decide who will write the final report of the SAT for review by the Advocacy Committee, the Board, and the annual Program Evaluation Committee of the Advocacy Committee. (See Chapter Eight for discussion of the latter). The report can be written by the staff advocate, the chairperson or an SAT member.

The people in the final meeting or the writer, if no meeting is possible, can use the Guide for Writing the Annual (or Final) Report of the Study Action Team set forth in Figure 7 and the Final Action Planning form (see Figure 6 in Chapter Six) to pull together both measurable and non-measurable results as well as those that were not achievable. Answers to the questions regarding results will give the SAT's evaluation of its work. Narrative comments concerning the questions will enhance the report.

If it is not possible to have a final celebration and evaluation meeting, send a letter of thanks to the total advocacy group (even those who may have dropped out along the way) and a copy of the final SAT report.

In the next chapter we will focus on how to do an annual evaluation of each SAT and the total advocacy program.

EXERCISE

This exercise is a follow-up to the study-action planning exercise in Chapter Six. Use the Action Plan arrived at for that advocacy problem (the one in the log or your own) to practice taking action.

Divide into three groups and role play. Groups should be no smaller than three and no larger than seven. In each advocate group exercise, have members take certain roles: host, lead presenter, assistant presenters, resource persons, notetakers, observers, and any other roles that seem needed. Think about special skills needed from these people. Who is ready to be a diplomat? Who is comfortable with confrontation? Who "teaches" well? Agree who will use these skills.

Group I: Assume that the decision-makers are in essential agreement with the change and, when they understand the problem, are likely to work with you to make the necessary changes or provide a new program. Use dialogue as your intervention.

Group II: Assume that some of the decision-makers will agree and some will disagree, so that you will have to educate and negotiate in order to intervene successfully.

<u>Group III</u>: Assume that the decision-makers are in major disagreement. Use all levels of intervention as needed, up to and including <u>confrontation</u>.

This exercise can be extended and enriched if there are parallel groups of decision-makers who will talk with each group. There should be a decision-makers group to talk with Group I who are essentially in agreement, a group to talk with Group II where some of the decision-makers are in agreement and some are not, and a group to work with Group III where most of the decision-makers are in major disagreement. Give the latter different roles appropriate to their system.

If possible, two people who are not decision-makers or advocates should be given the role of outside observers of each group meeting.

Use one-third of the time to prepare for the meeting, one-third to talk together, and one-third to debrief.

<u>Debriefing</u>: Have decision-makers discuss how they felt about the approach of the advocates: what was helpful? what was not? Have advocates critique themselves and discuss what they learned. Finally, ask the observers to grade the advocates on the adequacy of their advocacy skills and provide constructive criticism regarding what they did well and what they could have done better.

This exercise works well in a one day workshop or in a class period for students where it can follow the earlier study-action planning exercise. (See Chapter Six).

REFERENCES

BIKLEN, D. (1974) Let Our Children Go. Syracuse: Human Policy Press.

BRAGER. G. and H. SPECHT (1973) Community Organizing. New York: Columbia.

SUNLEY, R. (1970) "Family Advocacy: From Case to Cause." Social Casework (June) 351.

EIGHT

EVALUATION

Evaluation of advocacy work as it progresses has been stressed throughout our discussion. It is therefore essential to do an annual evaluative overview of your advocacy program and its component parts: SAT's, coalitions, legislative lobbying, position papers and so forth.

IMPORTANCE OF EVALUATION

An annual evaluation is important for these reasons: first, it provides accountability and visibility at all levels: administration, board, staff, funding sources, the community and accreditation bodies. Second, it provides perspective on the effectiveness of organization, process and results. Third, it enables administrative staff, the Advocacy Committee and the Board to look back in order to plan for the future: to allocate staff and volunteer time and to improve cost-effectiveness. Fourth, evaluation findings can be shared with funding sources, the community or accreditation bodies to improve their awareness of your advocacy work.

In this chapter we will look at how various levels of evaluation -- from those that are very subjective to those that are reasonably objective -- can be done, how a systematic evaluation process can be developed and finally, how the evaluation results can be used.

Let me say here that all this talk about how important it is to evaluate should not intimidate you. Evaluation is merely looking back at what you have done in a systematic way, measured against ideas of what should happen. At first, you may use a very subjective evaluation of how well or poorly your program worked measured against norms in the heads of those commenting on the program. Later, when your program has become more established, you could develop a more objective evaluation based on measurable objectives and accurate statistical information. You can then measure the program's results against the objectives set for it. Let us examine the various levels of evaluation from one that is largely subjective to one that is more objective.

The easiest evaluation is one that is based on narrative reports and arrives at an impression of what has been done well, what needs to be improved and what particular efforts have failed. This type of evaluation is, of course, the least objective and most prone to reflect the biases of the evaluators. It is, however, a beginning and can be a base from which to learn from both success and failure. Bias can be reduced somewhat by having the advocacy coordinator and the Advocacy Committee read and evaluate annual reports of advocacy work. An Advocacy Committee meeting could be set aside to discuss each person's findings.

The next level of objectivity in evaluation is one in which you might try to pull together whatever statistics you have collected about the program to substantiate and enlarge the impressionistic evaluation. These statistics might include: the number of SAT's that were active in that year, the number of people served, the number of meetings held to achieve the results, the hours of staff and volunteer time used, the dollars brought to the agency as a result of advocacy work and the referrals to other agency programs as a result of your work in advocacy or your visibility in the community.

The most objective and also the most difficult evaluation is based on the systematic collection of data regarding component parts of the advocacy program, which are then evaluated against the objectives set at the beginning of the year. Wherever possible these objectives should be measurable. These can be compared with the actual results at the end of the year.

Let us assume that you want to do the best evaluation that you can within the limitations of the agency's capability. Some agencies have computerized statistics and an elaborate planning process. Other agencies may plan and evaluate all programs on a subjective basis with minimal statistical information. In your situation what will you need to have in place in order to evaluate your advocacy program and its component parts as objectively as possible? Where can you begin and what else might you need to do to extend your evaluative effectiveness?

At the beginning of the chapter we looked at why we need to do an evaluation and for whom we do it. Now, let us examine the aspects that you will need to consider to develop a systematic evaluation process: what do you want to evaluate and how frequently? What are the goals and objectives that will form a base from which to evaluate advocacy efforts? How can you develop guidelines from which to evaluate your advocacy program? How can you develop an information base from which to evaluate? Who will do the evaluation and how will they do it? How will the evaluation results be used? Let us look at each of these aspects more carefully.

WHAT DO YOU WANT TO EVALUATE AND HOW FREQUENTLY?

No doubt you will want to evaluate your advocacy program annually. To evaluate your overall advocacy program you will need to consider: whether the program as executed is in conformance to the goals set for it; whether the process by which the goals were met proceeded adequately; and, whether the program is worth doing in terms of the results achieved. Similar questions will need to be asked to evaluate the parts of the program: SAT's, coalitions, lobbying, and so forth. For the purposes of our discussion here, let us look first at evaluation of the program and then, using the SAT as the main vehicle in advocacy work, look at the evaluation of an SAT.

WHAT ARE THE GOALS AND OBJECTIVES THAT WILL FORM THE BASE FROM WHICH YOU WILL EVALUATE ADVOCACY EFFORTS?

Every evaluation must have a base from which to evaluate. An advocacy program's base is rooted in the goals and objectives set out for the program. In turn, the advocacy program itself is derived from the agency's objectives, which are rooted in the agency's overall goals and objectives. The agency's goals and objectives are in turn developed from the agency's purpose or charter (See Figure 8). Think of the evaluation process as circular. It begins with what you hoped to do (your goal) and sets specific objectives. When the work is done, it looks at how well or how poorly you did the work and to what extent you reached your goal and objectives.

To develop your own advocacy program goals and objectives from which to evaluate refer to Figure 8 and the goals and objectives as formulated by another agency in Chapter Four, then look at the information you have in your own agency.

1. Look up the written purpose or charter of your agency.

2. If your agency has gone through a planning process, look up the goals and objectives that have been set forth to carry out the agency's work.

3. Write down the specific goals calling for advocacy work.

4. Write down the overall goal of your advocacy program. (You should be able to get this from your original definition of what advocacy was to be in your agency.) Compare 3 and 4 and make sure the advocacy program goal carries out the agency goals relating to advocacy.

124

THE PROCESS OF ADVOCACY PROGRAM EVALUATION

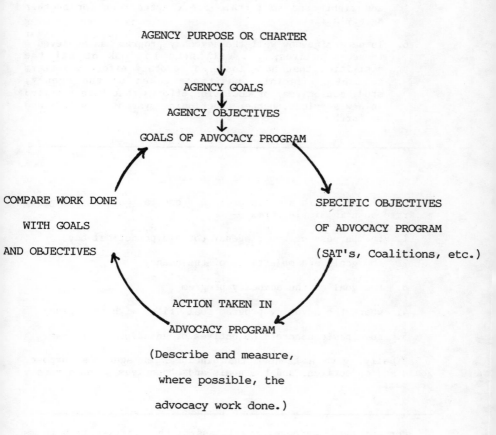

FIGURE 8

5. Now, think through the basic objectives of your advocacy program. These are much more detailed and will include the various aspects of advocacy in which you feel you must be involved in your community. (You might include: identifying unmet needs or rights, changing dysfunctional systems, creating new services, educating regarding needs and rights and so forth. See Chapter Four for another agency's list.)

6. To determine how well the advocacy program has achieved those objectives, you will need to look at all the activities that have fostered advocacy efforts: letters to public officials, positions taken by the agency, study-action team or coalition efforts that have resulted in new services, better functioning systems, new laws and so forth.

Optional Exercise

As an exercise in a class or in a presentation, ask the group to write down in simple terms --

1. the purpose of their agency (or a hypothetical one)

2. the goals and objectives of the agency

3. the goal of the advocacy program

4. where the advocacy program goal "fits" with the agency

5. some basic concrete objectives of an advocacy program.

Finally, give a handout that includes an agency's purpose, goals and objectives, and the goals and objectives of an advocacy program.

For our purposes here, I will assume that study-action teams (coalitions or committees) will be the major vehicles for advocacy work. Think through how you will evaluate an SAT. This is really a similar process: look at the goals and objectives of the advocacy program (See Figure 9). Does the SAT carry out those goals and objectives? Which? In evaluating an SAT you will want to look at its goals and objectives compared to the results it achieved. You will also want to look at how well the SAT was organized and how well the study and action process was carried out. In addition, you will want to evaluate the results -- both the quantity and the quality of the work.

126

THE PROCESS OF STUDY-ACTION TEAM EVALUATION

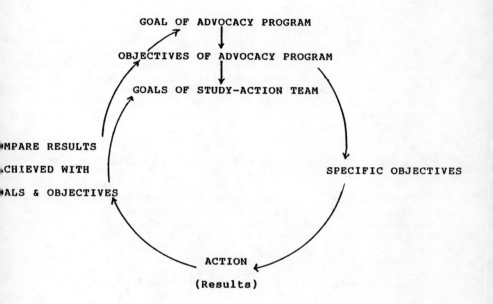

FIGURE 9

127

We will look now at how to develop detailed guidelines for evaluation of advocacy work.

HOW CAN YOU DEVELOP GUIDES FROM WHICH TO EVALUATE YOUR ADVOCACY PROGRAM

It will be necessary, of course, to develop two sets of evaluation guides: one for overall program evaluation and one for evaluating each aspect of advocacy work. Since the study-action team has been the major vehicle for advocacy work considered here, we will look at how to develop a guide for evaluating the SAT. Such a guide could be adapted easily to evaluation of task forces, coalitions, legislative lobbying and so forth. Let us begin with the particular (SAT's) and move to the general (program) later.

GUIDE FOR ANNUAL (OR FINAL) EVALUATION OF A STUDY-ACTION TEAM

Evaluation questions for an SAT in process or that has ended are really similar to those asked at the end of the study phase or the action planning phase. (Compare Figure 4: Guide for Evaluation of a Study-Action Team). Added now is additional information about results and the overall effort. There is an attempt also to assess significance and to give an overall rating. The following questions are useful as a guide for SAT evaluation annually or at the time of the final report.

Conformance to Goals

Does the initial charge to the SAT (and/or the current goal) match the goals of the agency and the Advocacy Program?

Which objectives of the Advocacy Program are addressed by the SAT?

Organization

Is the SAT operating within a well-defined charge (original or new)?

Are estimates to complete the work realistic re: people to be served, time frames, number of meetings, staff and volunteers needed?

Should the SAT be reorganized in any way?

Process

Analysis

Is there clear analysis of the problem, the proposed solution and the system within which the SAT seeks change?

Goals and Objectives

Are the SAT's goals and objectives clear?

Action Plan

Are there specific action objectives to carry out the goal?

If action objectives are planned, are they achievable?

Is the intervention plan appropriate to the task/situation?

Advocacy Resources

Are the needed advocacy resources available: documentation, power base, technical expertise, facilitating skills, funding?

Results

Were the action objectives to carry out the goal achieved?

Was the SAT's goal achieved?

Were the estimates of people to be served, time frames, staff and volunteers needed for completion of the work appropriate in terms of actual results?

Were the measurable results significant?

Were non-measurable results significant?

Were secondary gains valuable for the agency? for the community?

Were the results worth the effort and cost required?

Was the process well done even if results were poor or nil?

How was the advocacy effort perceived by the people served?

Rating

Give a rating to each question in the guidelines according to the rating scale below, then give an overall rating to the

SAT (not a mathematical total). For each aspect, give reasons for the rating, particularly if it is low, and add any questions or comments. Indicate your subjective comments regarding the quality of the advocacy work and the results. What could have improved the overall results of the SAT?

Rating Scale: 0-1 Unacceptable   2 - Fair   3 - Good
              4 Excellent   5 - Outstanding

GUIDE FOR ANNUAL EVALUATION OF THE ADVOCACY PROGRAM

To design a guide for program evaluation, think about what it is you want to review. Is the advocacy work that is being done in conformance with the agency's and the advocacy program's goals and objectives? Is the process of orienting and involving board and staff members, choosing issues, establishing and monitoring SAT's proceeding adequately? Is there an ongoing evaluation of the advocacy program and process? Are the results significant in terms of quantity and quality? Information to answer these questions should be found in the Annual Report of the Advocacy Program compiled by the advocacy coordinator and from the experience of the Advocacy Committee.

The following guide is an example of how these can be detailed. Your program may need additional or different questions.

Conformance to Goals

Does the current work of the Advocacy Committee effectively address the goals and objectives of the agency and the Advocacy Program?

Are all goals and objectives receiving an appropriate amount of attention.

Process

Orienting and Involving Board and Staff

Is the Advocacy Committee encouraging awareness of the Advocacy Program among staff and board members?

Are staff and board encouraged to participate in the Advocacy Program by logging issues and working on SAT'?

Choosing Issues

Are logs being presented to the Committee in a timely manner?

Do the logs contain sufficient data for decision-making purposes?

Is the Committee able to select or reject issues appropriately? (See Criteria for Choosing Issues in Chapter Five.)

Does the Committee see that the Advocacy Program structure is followed? (See Flow of Issues.)

Establishing SATs

Is the Committee making sure that the charge to an SAT is reasonable in scope and clarity?

Are people who have experienced the problem for which an SAT is established involved in the advocacy process whenever possible?

Are SATs established in a reasonable amount of time?

Are SATs established and organized in a manner that allows them to operate in an effective and efficient manner?

Monitoring SATs

Are ongoing SATs adequately monitored and kept on track?

Does the Committee suggest ways to restructure, refocus, or reorganize SATs if needed?

Evaluating the Advocacy Program and Process

Are there open and effective channels of communication between the Advocacy Committee and the board?

Does the Committee evaluate and consider means to improve the quality of the advocacy process and the overall program on an ongoing basis?

Are resources (staff, volunteers, clerical time and supplies) being used appropriately?

Are agency, staff and board properly utilized re: input on logs? involvement in SATs? communication of current activity?

Results

Actual Results

Compare the following to the last three years:

131

How many logs were filed?

How many SAT's were started?

How many SAT's were active, inactive, or waiting?

How many SAT's were completed?

How many people (staff, board, Advocacy Committee, community) were involved in SAT's?

How many resource people were contacted to provide expertise for the SAT?

How many people were impacted by SAT's: directly? indirectly?

Is the Advocacy Program's use of SAT's as the primary vehicle for advocacy work getting the expected results? If not, why not?

Significance of Results

Cost Effectiveness

How many person hours were spent on advocacy: (board, staff, Advocacy Committee, community)?

What is the annual cost of the Advocacy Program?

What is the per hour cost of the program: (professional, clerical, and overhead)?

What is the per hour cost of the program per person served?

What income was produced by the Advocacy Program?

Is the work done by the Advocacy Program cost effective?

Qualitative Effectiveness

Much that is done in advocacy is non-measurable; from a qualitative standpoint, is the work done by the Advocacy Program worth doing?

HOW CAN YOU DEVELOP AN INFORMATION BASE
FROM WHICH TO EVALUATE?

To evaluate effectively it is vital to build in an

information base that will tell you how well you have achieved the goals and objectives of the advocacy program and those of each issue. Just as a counseling program is expected to keep statistics and records, an advocacy program needs similar expectations. You will need an information base of narrative reports of advocacy activities and statistics on various aspects that can be compiled in an annual report. Let us look at what the information base for an advocacy program should be.

NARRATIVE REPORTS

Advocacy Committee minutes provide the narrative record of what the program has dealt with over the year: logs reviewed, SAT's set up, charges to SAT's, recommendations regarding action planning of given SAT's, positions taken re legislative and other issues, ad hoc committees set up to deal with advocacy process issues, decisions made about process issues and termination of SAT's. This may be only a partial list.

The advocacy record or file should contain the log, a face sheet, minutes, the initial report of study, interim reports, the final action plan and reports of changes in focus or action plans as discussed in Chapter Five.

The Guide for Writing the Annual (or Final) Report of the Study-Action Team shown in Figure 7 (See Chapter Seven) can be used to pull together the information to date on the SAT's work for an annual (or final) report. This information combined with the projected and actual measures in the Final Action Planning form (see Chapter Six) will provide a clear view of the problem, the SAT's goals and objectives and what has or has not been achieved. Minutes and statistics of SAT activities are additional sources of information for the staff advocate who prepares the annual report. Note that the Guide (Figure 7) asks for the SAT's subjective evaluation of its efforts as well as asking for as much that is measurable as possible since a qualitative as well as quantitative assessment is needed. Narrative comments regarding certain aspects will enhance understanding of the SAT's work that are not fully explained by numbers.

STATISTICAL REPORTS

Build in statistical reporting after each SAT meeting with an SAT meeting data sheet. This sheet should seek at least the following information: the meeting date, the number of staff hours and volunteer hours spent in the SAT meetings, the number of people served directly and as collaterals (adults, children, male, female, ethnic origin). This information can be gathered by the staff advocate on the SAT data sheet at each meeting and given to the statistician. Where appropriate, data can be noted regarding the way advocacy work is affecting the agency in other ways: referrals to other programs such as counseling or family life education, publicity through TV presentations and newspaper articles, and fees earned by the SAT for consultation, workshops, presentations or other efforts. (See SAT Meeting Data Sheet in Appendix 4.) These data can be compiled on a monthly, quarterly or annual basis by the statistician (or the staff advocate, if the agency has little statistical help); data regarding the number of SAT's, their status (active, waiting to be formed, inactive, terminated), number of meetings held, number of people served, number of staff and volunteer hours expended can be available for the Board, Advocacy Committee and agency planning committees to review as the year progresses.

Daily statistical report sheets in some agencies record time spent in direct or indirect service (preparation or administration) in a given program. It is useful in advocacy to be able to record direct service such as meetings of SAT's, conferences with chairpersons or action meetings with system people, workshops, lobbying legislators and so forth. A record of time spent in indirect service is useful also to show the ratio of preparation time to direct advocacy activity. This is usually much higher in advocacy work than in counseling, for example. These service statistics are helpful in indicating staff time used in the program. They form a basis from which to evaluate the past year's use of staff time and to plan the allocation of staff time for the following year. The executive director can supply the Advocacy Program cost and breakdown in terms of personnel costs (professional and clerical) and costs of supplies and overhead.

ANNUAL REPORT

An annual report of the Advocacy Program should be compiled by the advocacy coordinator. This should include all of the SAT annual reports, a summary of the year's accomplishments and tables and narrative that review the year's work. The report should also answer questions in the Guide for Annual Evaluation of the Advocacy Program. Some suggested items are: a table indicating the new issues that were logged, their disposition and the charge to the SAT's, if they were set up; a table indicating the names of active, inactive, waiting, or terminated SAT's for the current year and their projected status and time needs for the following year; a table indicating a summary of the advocacy program statistics: new issues logged, study action teams, legislative activity (positions and letters), number of advocates working in the program (staff, board and community volunteers).

There should be a table indicating in what way each SAT served people and the number of people (adult, child, male, female, and ethnic origin) served by advocacy and/or referred to other agency programs; a table summarizing the advocacy statistics by each study-action team; number of meetings;

volunteers and staff used; number of hours spent in meetings by volunteers and staff; number of resource people contacted (those whose opinion, advice or expertise was sought in the study phase); number of people served (adults, children, and ethnic origin) number of referrals to other agency programs, number of dollars brought to the agency by advocacy work; a table to show comparison with the three previous years of the number of new logs filed; new SAT's begun; SAT's active in the year; SAT's inactive; SAT's completed; staff (and students), board and community people involved, hours spent on advocacy (staff, Board, Advocacy Committee, community) and people served.

It is important to set forth the annual cost of the program, the per hour cost (personnel and overhead) and the per hour cost per person served. Subtract from the cost of the program any income produced by advocacy work. The per hour cost per person served is a very uncertain computation because so many people are served in advocacy efforts of whom we are not aware statistically, for instance, where TV or newspapers are involved. For this reason a narrative should answer questions on the significance of results in cost effectiveness and qualitative effectiveness.

WHO WILL DO THE EVALUATION AND HOW WILL THEY DO IT?

To my mind, evaluation can be done best by an ad hoc Advocacy Program Evaluation Committee made up of board members, professionals outside the agency, persons who have experienced a problem about which you have advocated, and a staff advocate-- all of whom have worked on SAT's and are, or have been, active on the Advocacy Committee. (Objectivity for the current year is gained if several are no longer actively working in advocacy but are familiar with the process.) In addition, the Advocacy Committee chairperson, the advocacy coordinator and the executive director or the director of professional services should be on the Program Evaluation Committee. This committee need not be too large, possibly eight people.

Committee members should have a guide to evaluation packet that includes: agency goals related to advocacy, a definition of the goal of the advocacy program, advocacy program objectives, criteria for choosing issues, guide for annual (or final) evaluation of an SAT and guide for annual evaluation of the advocacy program. In addition, each evaluator should be given one copy of the guide for evaluation of each SAT to be read. As the evaluator reads, she/he can include their comments or questions, rate each aspect and give a final rating. It is important that the evaluator give reasons for the rating of each aspect, particularly if the rating is low, and include subjective comments regarding the quality of the advocacy work and the results.

A secretary should be chosen from the Program Evaluation Committee, or a person from the clerical or professional staff added to the committee for this important function. The secretary should note the ratings of each SAT after it is reviewed. Additional narrative comments to elaborate on the Program Evaluation Committee's findings will be needed.

The Program Evaluation Committee can use the annual Advocacy Program Report as its major information base. The Annual Report will include reports on all SAT's and statistical tables relating to the program. Additional information can be sought from SAT chairpersons or members as needed.

The Advocacy Committee chairperson should chair the Program Evaluation Committee. She/he and the advocacy coordinator should divide up the work into two or three parts and send only the part of the work for each evaluation meeting about ten days ahead. This prevents members feeling overwhelmed with their task and promotes concentration on a specific piece. By the last meeting of the committee the full annual report should be in their hands. To aid in evaluation it is especially valuable to get feedback from people served through advocacy efforts. People who were served by a new service can be polled and their comments quoted. Evaluation forms can gain feedback from workshop participants or specific presentations. Impressions gained from comments of people over the year can be included. However, much of what advocacy does cannot be measured, or its benefits made known to the advocates.

In evaluation of advocacy work, measurable results are usually just the tip of the iceberg. How do you measure the impact of suicide prevention courses in schools that promote open discussion of how to deal with stress and prevent suicide? How do you measure the value of workshops for clergy, guidance counselors and teachers on what it feels like to be a child of divorce? Can you measure the value of reduced alienation of spouses using the no-fault divorce law or the value of the custody law that encourages the continuing involvement of both parents in parenting. Obviously, many advocacy interventions, although extremely valuable, are not measurable. Whether it is educating, trying to change a dysfunctional system, lobbying for passage of a law or setting up a new service, advocacy works on broad issues with multiple ramifications for change about which we may never know.

An advocacy program evaluation will take several hours: it can be done in one day (or part of a day) at some spot away from the agency, or in two or three two-hour committee meetings. Be sure to set a definite time frame for completion of the evaluation. Findings and recommendations of the Program Evaluation Committee should be added to the annual report and the whole presented to the Advocacy Committee for their review prior to the Board's review.

HOW WILL THE EVALUATION RESULTS BE USED?

Evaluation results will be used primarily by an agency's own administrators (the executive, the director of professional services and the advocacy coordinator), the Advocacy Committee and the Board of Directors to assess the quality and quantity of advocacy work and its cost effectiveness.

The evaluation findings can be used by the administration to plan staff deployment for the following year and to set objectives for time use in the Advocacy Program. For example, how many SAT's you take on will depend on staff time allocated. However, some SAT's take longer than others and it is often difficult to know the length of time needed when you begin to work on an issue. This is similar to the difficulty in setting objectives in counseling where it is hard to know how long a "case" may need. In spite of this, administrators have set measurable objectives for counseling and we can do this as well for advocacy.

If time frames are set for the study and action phases of SAT's this will give the executive, the advocacy coordinator and the Advocacy Committee a better idea of how long each SAT will take. An estimate can then be made of the number of SAT's that could be taken on in the next year. This can be refined a little further by looking at those SAT's that will be active in the coming year (needing monthly or twice-monthly meetings) and those that will be less active or inactive (for example, waiting for legislation to move). Of course, the retrospective look at the previous year's work and the time frames needed will be valuable also in making projections for the coming year.

In your agency, you could use evaluation findings and yearly program statistics to help to make projections for your future work. You might feel that you have an outside limit of two or four SAT's that you could work on in one year. If some turn out to be short-term, you could do more; if some are long-term, that will be your effort over several years. At times some SAT's may have to be put on hold while you deal with some urgent issue that has immediate consequences for your clients and other families in the community.

Evaluation should give insights into where the process or management of advocacy work needs to be improved. Does the Advocacy Committee need to improve its selection of issues, or the way it limits the charge to a given SAT? Is there a way to do more advocacy with the staff and volunteer time available? Is the program serving enough people to justify its continuance? Is the Advocacy Program enhancing other agency programs and the agency's visibility in the community?

137

Evaluation findings can make good public relations material for the agency, not only because of the people served, but because of advocacy's cooperative work with other organizations in the community. In addition, effective evaluations can be used to justify continuance of funding as well as to increase awareness of how previous funds were used. Evaluation results will be needed increasingly as more and more cities and counties in the United States develop overall planning of both public and private human services. Evaluation information could be used effectively to testify on behalf of needed programs at the state and federal level, whether for generic advocacy programs or specific programs for unmet needs based on the findings of certain SAT's.

These findings can be used internally as well to educate board, staff and other community volunteers regarding the efficacy of advocacy work.

You may feel after reading this: "How can our organization ever do all this; convince the board to set up a program, find funding, recruit volunteers, decide on issues, then work on them? Finally, you ask us to go back and evaluate everything that we have done!"

You can do it! Take it step by step. Do your homework-- whether it is convincing your board that advocacy is a needed service or convincing a funding body that a new service is essential in your community. If you can, begin with some issue with which you have a good chance of success. Gradually take on issues as you have time and enthusiastic advocates to work on them. Your skills will increase as you work together. Encourage your program to grow as staff and funds permit. Look frequently at what would make your program better. Evaluation -- at whatever level -- helps you to do this. Good luck!

DEFINITION OF FAMILY ADVOCACY BY THE FAMILY ADVOCACY NETWORK*

"Family Advocacy as practiced in a Family Service Agency is a service directed to improving conditions for families by harnessing expert knowledge of family needs with the commitment to action and the skills to produce necessary change. It involves a process of working in alliance with or/on behalf of a family or individual, a group of families, a neighborhood, or a community, to develop strategies for changing institutionalized conditions, systems, or administrative practices that are seen to have a negative effect on individuals and family life. Family Advocacy goals include not only improvement of existing public and voluntary services and their delivery, but also provision of new or changed forms of social utilities. Specific objectives may change as client groups develop capacity for self-reliant action in regard to one problem or interest and move to others that require service. Family advocacy refers to cause advocacy. It is expected that Family Service practitioners carry out individual case advocacy as an established aspect of all family practice, conceiving of it as part of their social casework or family life education/development/enrichment practice. As these case advocacy activities prove to reflect neighborhood, community, State, and National problems, they become part of the information base an agency uses in its advocacy program." (Based on FSAA definition, 1971, and FSAA Staff Position Paper, 1978.)

September, 1978

---

*The Family Advocacy Network is an organization of advocates (staff, board and executives of family agencies) in FSAA member agencies whose purpose is to educate, support and encourage advocacy in member agencies.

ADVOCACY LOG

FAMILY AND CHILDREN'S SERVICE
    OF LANCASTER COUNTY, PA

DATE _____ , 19

LOG NO. _____

CASE NO. _____

LOGGED BY _____

SYSTEMS DYSFUNCTION

UNMET NEEDS
(Gaps in Service)

Care of Aged ____	Mental Health ____	
Child Care ____	Phys. Health ____	
Corrections ____	Pub. Assist. ____	
Education ____	Public Safety ____	
Employment ____	Recreation ____	
Housing ____	Social Serv. ____	
Internal ____	Transport. ____	
Legal ____	Other (specify) ____	

_____

_____

UNMET RIGHTS

_____

_____

CASE SITUATION

    Problem:

    Action taken (or attempted) within system:

ADVOCACY PROBLEM (brief statement) Who hurts? Why?

PROBLEM ANALYSIS*

    Documentation: No. affected _____   Not known _____

                      How widespread? (local, state, national)

                      To what degree affected? _____

                      Who else can help document? _____

    Legal and social context: (Laws and regulations under which system
                                    operates)

                    Legal/moral rights of persons involved:

SOLUTION ANALYSIS

    What change is necessary?

             What would be a better way to handle problem?

             What would success look like? from professional viewpoint?
             from clients' viewpoint?

             $ needed _____? volunteers _____

    Who can make the change(s) necessary?

             Key decision-maker(s) _____

             Within system—forces of opposition_____

                              forces of support_____

             Who on the "inside" can help us understand the system and/or
             influence it?

    Who will support us in work on this issue?

    Who will oppose?

*Fill in all of the information that you can. If a Study-Action Team is
established, they will look into these areas in greater detail.

FACESHEET FOR STUDY-ACTION TEAM

Name of SAT_____ Log No. _____

Chairperson_____ Date of Log_____

Date of Initial Meeting _____

STUDY PHASE

Charge to the SAT as approved by Board on _____)

Time frame:

Changes in the Charge during the Study Phase:

Time frame:

ACTION PHASE

Action Plan (as approved by Board on _____)

Time frame:

Changes in the Action Plan:

Time frame:

SAT ENDED

Date _____

FACESHEET (continued)
Page 2

Participants

NAME   ADDRESS   PHONE

143

SAT MEETING DATA SHEET

NAME _____ DATE _____

CHAIRPERSON_____ STAFF ADVOCATE_____

SAT MEMBERS

	No.	Hrs.	Total
Volunteers	_____	_____	_____
Staff	_____	_____	_____

NAMES OF RESOURCE PEOPLE[1]

_____   _____

_____   _____

SINCE LAST MEETING

	Adults M F Eth.[4]	Children M F Eth.	How Served
No. of People Served Directly[2]	_____	_____	_____
No. of Collaterals Served[3]	_____	_____	_____
Impact of Advocacy on the Agency:			
Referrals to Counseling	_____	_____	_____
Referrals to FLE	_____	_____	_____
Increased Awareness of the Agency:	_____	_____	_____

$$ earned by the SAT (fees, contracts, honoraria, etc.)

	$$	To or For
Consultation	_____	_____
Workshops	_____	_____
Presentations	_____	_____
Other	_____	_____

[1]People from whom SAT members seek consultation or information to further the work of the study and action phases of advocacy work, for example, legislators, administrators, etc.

[2]People who are experiencing the problem for whom a program is developed to meet their previously unmet need.

[3]People who will, if their consciousness is raised, or their skills increased, serve their constituents in a new or better way.

[4]Ethnic: W—White; B—Black; H—Hispanic: O—Other

SPECIALIZED LITIGATION AND SUPPORT CENTERS
AS RESOURCES FOR ADVOCATES*

The following litigation and support centers are funded by the Legal
Corporation except those marked **.

**American Civil Liberties Union
84 Fifth Avenue
New York, NY   10011
(212) 944-9800

Center for Law and Education
6 Appian Way, Gutman Library, 3rd Fl.
Harvard University, Cambridge, Mass.
(617) 495-4666

**Center for Law & Social Policy
1751 N Street, NW
Washington, D.C.
(202) 872-0670

Center on Social Welfare Policy and Law
95 Madison Avenue, Room 701
New York, NY   10016
(212) 679-3709

Children's Defense Fund
1520 New Hampshire Ave., NW
Washington, D.C.   20036
(202) 483-1470

Disability Rights Education & Defense Fund
2032 San Pablo Ave.
Berkeley, CA
(415) 644-2555

Education Law Center, Inc.
Philadelphia, PA   19102
(215) 732-6655

**Food Research and Action Center (FRAC)
1319 F St., NW, Suite 500
Washington, D.C.   20004
(202) 393-5060

Handicapped Persons Legal Support Unit
335 Broadway, Room 803
New York, NY   10013
(212) 925-1000

Indian Law Support Center, Native
American Rights Fund
1506 Broadway
Boulder, CO   80302
(303) 447-8760

* Partial list

**Mental Disability Legal Resource Center
ABA, 1800 M St., NW
Washington, D.C. 20036
(202) 331-2240

Mental Health Law Project
2021 L St., NW, 8th Fl.
Washington, D.C. 20036
(202) 467-5730

Migrant Legal Action Program
806 Fifteenth St., NW, Suite 600
Washington, D.C. 20005
(202) 347-5100

National Center for Immigrants' Rights
1550 W. Eighth St.
Los Angeles, CA 90017
(213) 487-2531

National Center on Women & Family Law
799 Broadway, Room 402
New York, NY 10003
(212) 674-8200

National Center for Youth Law
1663 Mission St., 5th Fl.
San Francisco, CA 94103
(415) 543-3307

National Consumer Law Center
11 Beacon St., Suite 925
Boston, MA 02108
(617) 523-8010

National Economic Development & Law Center
2150 Shattuck Ave., Suite 300
Berkeley, CA 94704
(415) 548-2600

National Employment Law Project
475 Riverside Dr., Suite 240
New York, NY 10027
(212) 870-2121

---

236 Massachusetts Ave., NE
Washington, D.C. 20002
(202) 544-2185
(For current legislation & regulatory
matters only.)

National Health Law Program
2639 S. La Cienega Blvd.
Los Angeles, CA 90034
(213) 204-6010

National Housing Law Project
2150 Shattuck Ave., Suite 300
Berkeley, CA 94704
(415) 548-9400

146

**National Legal Aid and Defender Association
1625 K St., NW, Suite 800
Washington, D.C. 20006
(202) 452-0620

NLADA Access to Justice Project
Same address and phone number

National Senior Citizens Law Center
1636 W. Eighth St., Suite 201
Los Angeles, CA   90017
(213) 388-1381

National Social Science and Law Center
1825 Connecticut Ave., NW, Suite 401
Washington, D.C. 20009
(202) 797-1100

National Veterans Law Center
4900 Massachusetts Ave., NW
Washington, D.C.   20016
(202) 686-2741

APPENDIX 6

WORKSHEET FOR THE FIRST PHASE OF STUDY-ACTION PLANNING: PROBLEM, SOLUTION AND GOAL ANALYSIS

PROBLEM ANALYSIS

1. What is the problem? Who is hurting? Why? _____

2. How many are hurting? _____

3. What is the community, state or national attitude to the problem? _____

4. What is the attitude to the problem in the system where the problem occurs? _____

SOLUTION ANALYSIS

1. What change is needed? (alternative solutions) _____

2. What is the legal or moral basis for change? _____

3. Who has tried to solve this problem before? How? With what results? _____

4. What are the means to enable change? (Key decision-makers? Funds? Volunteers? Education? New law?) _____

5. What are the facilitating factors for change? (allies, funds, etc.) _____

What are the limiting factors? (Who or where is your opposition?) _____

6. What is the desired solution: the overall goal? _____

GOAL ANALYSIS

What are the objectives to carry out the goals:

Short term goal: maximum/minimum objectives? _____

Long term goal: maximum/minimum objectives? _____

148

WORKSHEET FOR THE SECOND PHASE OF STUDY: PLANNING STRATEGY FOR ACTION

GOAL: _____

ACTION OBJECTIVES: Short-Term Goal: Maximum Objectives _____
                   Long-Term Goal: Minimum Objectives _____
                   Estimate: Numbers to be Served _____ Time Frame _____

OUTLINE OF THE ADVOCACY CASE FOR CHANGE: (Problem definition, change needed, goals and objectives)

SYSTEM ANALYSIS
   WHO are the key decision makers who have power to make changes? _____
   WHO on the "inside" might help to understand the system? _____
   WHAT are some praiseworthy aspects of what they are doing? _____

   WHERE do the system's goals and objectives match those of the advocate group? _____

   WHERE do they differ? _____
   WHAT reaction can the advocate group expect: support?   resistance?   or a combination? _____

INTERVENTIONS
   WHERE will advocacy group intervene? _____
   HOW will the advocacy group intervene?   With what level of conflict: dialogue, education, negotiation,
      or confrontation?   With what tactics: letter, position paper, workshop, etc?
      (See Figure 5, Chapter Six)
   HOW will the advocacy group deal with resistance? _____
   WHO will do the intervening?   SAT?   Coalition?   People with the Problem? _____

EVALUATION OF THE STUDY-ACTION PLAN (See Guide for Evaluation of an SAT — Figure 4, Chapter Six)

FINAL ACTION PLANNING (See Figure 6 in Chapter Six)

   FINAL PREPARATION OF THE CASE FOR CHANGE

   Preparation for Initial Meeting with Key Decision-Makers:
   Meeting Place _____   Agenda _____
   Roles _____
   Preparation via training and role playing

ACTION PHASE

EVALUATION OF ACTION PHASE (See Guide to Final Evaluation of an SAT in Chapter Eight)

VERIFICATION OF CHANGE

TERMINATION

BIBLIOGRAPHY

ABERNATHY, J. (1976) "'76 Tax Reform Act Defines Guidelines for
    Lobbying by Tax-Exempt Organizations." Monitor.

AMBROSINO, S. (1976) "Integrating Counseling, Family Life Edu-
    cation, and Family Advocacy." Social Casework 60 (December):
    579-585.

ANSON, C. and ANDERSON, R. (1976) "The Art of Complaining." In
    Complaint Power." Maryland Center for Public Broadcasting.
    Owings Mills, Md.

BARRY, R.M. and MELUM, M.E. (1981) How to Follow Current Federal
    Legislation and Regulations. Report No. 81-197 C. Congres-
    sional Research Service. Washington, D.C.: Library of
    Congress.

BERLIN, I. (ed.) (1975) Advocacy for Child Mental Health. New
    York: Brunner/Mazel.

BIKLEN, D. (1973) "Power to Change." Syracuse University, Center
    on Human Policy. Unpublished paper.

BRAGER, G. (1968) "Advocacy and Political Behavior." Social Work
    13 (April)

BRAGER, G. and SPECHT, H. (1973) Community Organization. New
    York: Columbia University.

BRODY, R. and KRAILO, H. (1978) "An Approach to Reviewing the
    Effectiveness of Programs." Social Work 23.

CARLTON, T.O. and JUNG, M. (1972) "Adjustment Among Social Workers."
    Social Work (November)

CARNEGIE, D. (1936) How to Win Friends and Influence People.
    (CARNEGIE, D.D. and CARNEGIE, D. (eds.) (1981) Reprint Edi-
    tion, New York: Simon and Schuster.

COOPER, S. (1977) "Social Work: A Dissenting Profession." Social
    Work 22.

COX, F.M. et al. (1970) Strategies of Community Organization.
    Ithica, Ill: Peacock.

DEAN, W. (1977) "Back to Activism." Social Work 22.

DESCH, S. and TAYLOR, E. (1980) "Getting an Advocacy Program
    Started." Unpublished paper presented at Family Service
    Association of America Middle Atlantic Regional Council.

DLUHY, M.J. (1981) Changing the System. Beverly Hills: Sage.

DUDLEY, J.R. (1978) "Is Social Planning Social Work?" Social
Work 23.

FESSLER, D.R. (1976) Facilitating Community Change. La Jolla:
University Associates.

GARDNER, J.W. (1969) No Easy Victories. New York: Harper &
Row.

HAMBERG, J. et al. (1967) Where It's At: A Research Guide
for Community Organizing. Boston: New England Free Press.

HAMILTON, G. (1952) "The Role of Social Casework in Social
Policy." Social Casework 33 (October): 315-324.

HARTFORD, M.E. (1971) Groups in Social Work. New York: Columbia.

HARTMAN, A. (1974) "The Generic Stance and the Family Agency."
Social Casework (April).

KAHLE, J.H. (1970) "Relevant Agency Programs for the Large Urban
Community." Social Casework 51.

KAHN, A.J. (1969) Theory and Practice of Social Planning. New
York: Random House.

KAHN, A.,KAMMERMAN, S. and McGOWEN, B. (1972) Child Advocacy:
Report of a National Baseline Study. New York: Columbia
University School of Social Work.

KAMMERMAN, S. (1975) "A Paradigm for Programming: First Thoughts."
Social Service Review (September).

KATZ, D. and KAHN, R. (1966) The Social Psychology of Organizations. New York: John Wiley.

KIMMEL, W.A. (1977) Needs Assessment: A Critical Perspective.
Washington, D.C.:Dept. of Health, Education and Welfare.

LEVY, C.S. (1970) "The Social Worker as Agent of Policy Change."
Social Casework 51 (February): 102-108.

LIPPITT, G.L. (1973) Visualizing Change: Model Building and
the Change Process. La Jolla: University Associates.

LOURIE, N.V. (1970) "The Question of Advocacy: The Many Faces
of Advocacy." Public Welfare 30 (Spring): 12-15.

LURIE, E. (1970) How to Change the Schools. A Parent's Action
Handbook on How to Fight the System. New York: Random
House.

MALUCCIO, A.N. (1974) "Action as a Tool in Casework Practice."
Social Casework 55 (January): 30-35.

MANSER, E. (ed.)(1973) Family Advocacy: A Manual for Action.
New York: Family Service Association of America.

McCORMICK, M.J. (1970) "Social Advocacy: A New Dimension in Social Work." Social Casework 51: 3-10.

MENTAL HEALTH COMMUNITY INTERVENTION PROJECT (1975) Mastering Systems Intervention Skills: A Handbook for Community Mental Health and Family Service Professionals. Ann Arbor, Michigan: The University of Michigan.

NASW AD HOC COMMITTEE ON ADVOCACY (1969) "The Social Worker as Advocate: Champion of Social Victims." Social Work 14 (April):16-22.

NATIONAL ASSOCIATION OF SOCIAL WORKERS Code of Ethics as adopted by the 1979 Delegate Assembly, effective July 1, 1980.

NELSON, J. (1975) "Dealing with Resistance in Social Work Practice." Social Casework 56 (December): 587-592.

NEUBER, K.A. et al.(1980) Needs Assessment: A Model for Community Planning. Beverly Hills, Calif.: Sage.

O'CONNELL, B. (1978) "From Service to Advocacy to Empowerment." Social Casework (April).

PANITCH, A. (1974) "Advocacy in Practice." Social Work (May): 327.

PATTI, R. and RESNICK, H. (eds.) (1980) Change From Within: Humanizing Social Welfare Organizations. Philadelphia: Temple University Press.

PEARL, G. and BARR, D.H. (1976) "Agencies Advocating Together." Social Casework 57: 611- 618.

PRIGMORE, C. (1974) "Use of the Coalition in Legislative Action." Social Work 19 (January): 96-102.

REID, W.J. (1977) "Social Work for Social Problems." Social Work (September).

RICHAN, W.C. (1973) "Dilemmas of the Social Work Advocate." Child Welfare 52 (April): 220-226.

RICHAN, W.C. and ROSENBERG, M. (1971) The Advo-kit: A Self-administered Training Program for the Social Worker Advocate. Unpublished. Philadelphia: Temple University.

RILEY, P.V. (1971) "Family Advocacy: Case to Cause and Back to Case." Child Welfare (July).

ROBERTS, R.W. and NORTHEN, H. (eds.) (1976) Theories of Social Work with Groups. New York: Columbia.

ROTHMAN, J. (1974) Planning and Organizing for Social Change. New York: Columbia.

RYAN, W. (1976) Blaming the Victim. Random House.

SCHINDLER-RAINMAN, E. and LIPPITT, R. (1980) Building a Collaborative Community, Mobilizing Citizens for Action. Riverside: University of California Extension.

SCHWARTZ, W. (1976) in Theories of Social Work with Groups.
    Roberts, R.W. and Northen, H. (eds.) New York: Columbia.

SHERRY, P.H. (1970) "America's Third Force." Journal of Current
    Social Issues (July).

SOLOMON, B.B. (1976) Black Empowerment. New York: Columbia.

SUCHMAN, E.A. (1967) Evaluative Research. New York: Russell Sage.

SUNLEY, R. (1983) Advocating Today: A Human Service Practition-
    er's Handbook. New York: Family Service America.

SUNLEY, R. (1970) "Family Advocacy: From Case to Cause." Social
    Casework (June).

TAEBEL, D. (1972) "Strategies to Make Bureaucrats Responsive."
    Social Work 17 (November)

THE AD HOC COMMITTEE ON ADVOCACY (1969) "The Social Worker as
    Advocate: Champion of Social Victims." Social Work 14.

THURSZ, D. (1966) "Social Action as a Professional Responsibility."
    Social Work 11 (July): 12-21.

THURSZ, D. (1971) "The Arsenal of Social Action Strategies: Options
    for Social Workers." Social Work (January): 27-34.

WALTON, R. (1975) "Two Strategies of Social Change and Their
    Dilemmas." pp. 379-386 in Kramer and Specht (eds.)
    Readings in Community Organization Practice, Second Edition.
    Englewood Cliffs: Prentice Hall.

WASHBURN, B.J. (1976) "Lobbying by Public Charities: To Elect or
    Not to Elect." Tax Notes 4:3-12.

ABOUT THE AUTHOR

Eleanor Taylor was Advocacy Coordinator at Family Service of Lancaster County, PA from 1974 to 1990. She is currently an advocacy consultant.

A Master of Social Work graduate from the University of Toronto School of Social Work, Mrs. Taylor has had 34 years' experience in the social work field: in psychiatric, medical and family casework as well as in advocacy. She has made presentations and led workshops on advocacy at national and regional social work and family service conferences. In addition, she has taught casework and supervised field work for undergraduate social work students at Tunghai University in Taiwan and has been a visiting lecturer in undergraduate and graduate programs of social work in the United States.

A member of the National Association of Social Workers, she was also a member from 1983 to 1988 of the Council of Agency Professionals, an advisory group to the president and board of Family Service America (FSA). A member of the Pennsylvania Council of Family Agencies, she is formerly the co-chairperson of the Family Advocacy Network, Middle Atlantic Region of FSA.

Every two years FSA recognizes outstanding advocacy work by member agencies through the Margaret E. Rich Award and citations. In 1977 Family Service of Lancaster County was cited for its work in establishing a coalition that obtained a shelter for abused women in Lancaster. In 1981 the agency received the Rich Award for its work with systems affecting children of divorce.

In 1991 Mrs. Taylor was chosen Social Worker of the Year by the Central Region of the Pennsylvania National Association of Social Workers.